Medicinal & Poisonous Plants of India

Dr. C. ALAGESA BOOPATHI
Assistant Professor,
Department of Botany,
Government Arts College (Autonomous),
Salem – 636007,
Tamilnadu, India.

MJP
PUBLISHERS

ISBN 978-81-8094-285-3 **MJP Publishers**

Printed and bound in India

No. 47, Nallathambi Street,
Triplicane, Chennai 600 005

MJP 247

Publisher C. Janarthanan

Project Editor C. Ambica

To

My wife Sudha

&

Daughters Abarna and Arthi

PREFACE

India has rich diversity of medicinal and poisonous plants. About 90 percentage of herbal crude drugs useful in the manufacture of Siddha, Ayurveda, Unani, Homeopathy, Naturopathy, Amchi and Modern systems of medicine are widely from the wild source. This wild source is rapidly shrinking day-by-day. Therefore, there is a necessity for conservation and sustainable use of medicinal plants. Cultivation is clearly a sustainable possibility to the present collection of medicinal and poisonous plants from the wild. Medicinal plants yield numerous significance to the health of individual and communities. India is the largest producer of medicinal herbs and is appropriately called the botanical garden of the world.

Plants are the essential source of natural drugs. India is a country rich in indigenous herbal resources which grow on their varied topography and under changing agro climatic conditions permitting the growth of almost 20,000 plant species, of which about 2,500 are of medicinal importance. Plants which have one or more of its organs containing substances that can be used for the medicinal purpose are called medicinal plants. Medicinal plants are finding their way into pharmaceuticals, cosmetics and nutraceuticals. Plants have given western pharmacopoeia about 7,000 several pharmacologically important compounds and a number of top selling drugs of current times, e.g taxol, quinine, campothecine etc. Medicinal plants have been used as traditional treatments for numerous human diseases for thousands of years and in many parts of the world. As per World Health Organization estimates as many as 80 percentage of the world's population is still depending on traditional medicine as a source of the treatment of disease. In developing countries like India, 65 percentage of the population in the rural areas use traditional form of medicine to meet their prime healthcare necessities. Moreover, traditional medicine practices, which are conserved over decades from ancient civilizations, can serve as an effective assistance for the discovery and progress of current therapeutic drugs.

The medicinal utility of plants lies in some active chemical substances called phytochemicals that produce a definite physiological action on the human body. The phytochemicals are grouped into two main categories namely:

- Primary constituents which include amino acids, proteins, common sugars and chlorophyll etc., and
- Secondary plant metabolites consisting of alkaloids, flavonoids, tannins, essential oils, terpenoids, saponins, phenolic compounds, unsaturated sterols, triterpenoids etc.

Majority of phytochemicals have been known to possess valuable medicinal properties and some phytochemicals are toxic constituents. The plants thus find their medicinal importance due to respective phytoconstituents they contain. During the last few decades there has been an increasing interest in the research of medicinal plants and their traditional use in various parts of the world. There are considerable economic benefits in the development of indigenous medicines and in the use of medicinal plants for the treatment of various diseases. Natural products perform various functions and numerous of them have interesting and useful biological activities. Nature has bestowed on us a very rich botanical luxury and huge number of diverse types of plants grow in several parts of the country. Herbs do not exhibit instant treats, but rather offer a method to put the body in acceptable tune in nature. For many centuries, human have used herbs. Herbs have been used as medicines, as perfumes, as cosmetics, as flavours in foods, as disinfectants to preserve us against germs and as drugs to heal disorders.

This book provides information about more than 50 species of medicinal and poisonous plants with their photographs, scientific name, vernacular name, botanical description, distribution, propagation, plant parts used, phytochemical constituents, medicinal uses, toxic constituents, poisonous parts and poisonous symptoms.

I am extremely confident that this book will be useful to all the students, researchers and teachers in the field of medicinal plants.

I thank all my friends, colleagues, well-wishers, relatives and students for the constant encouragement to complete this work.

I am also thankful to P.Kadirvel and P.Janarthanan from Viva Computer, Salem-7 Institute for providing computer facility for typing and arranging figures in the manuscript.

I express my heartiest thanks and indebtedness to Mr.J.C. Pillai, Director of MJP Publishers, Chennai for his keen interest, encouragement and editorial efforts for publishing this book.

It is with great pleasure indeed that I dedicate the book to my father Mr.M.Chinnappan and my mother Mrs.C.Alamelu.

Valuable comments and suggestions from the readers are most welcome.

Dr. C. Alagesaboopathi

Table 1 List of Medicinal and Poisonous Plants

S.No.	Scientific Name	Family
1.	*Abrus precatorius* L.	Fabaceae
2.	*Abrus precatorius* L. (Black seed variety)	Fabaceae
3.	*Abrus precatorius* L. (Red seed variety)	Fabaceae
4.	*Abrus precatorius* L. (White seed variety)	Fabaceae
5.	*Abrus precatorius* L. (Yellow seed variety)	Fabaceae
6.	*Alangium salvifolium* (L.f.) Wangerin.	Alangiaceae
7.	*Annona squamosa* L.	Annonaceae
8.	*Argemone mexicana* L.	Papaveraceae
9.	*Calotropis gigentia* (L.) R.Br.	Asclepiadaceae
10.	*Calotropis procera* (Aiton) W.T. Aiton	Asclepiadaceae
11.	*Cannabis sativa* L.	Cannabinaceae
12.	*Carica papaya* L.	Caricaceae
13.	*Cascabela thevetia* (L.) Lippold	Apocynaceae
14.	*Cassia occidentalis* L.	Caesalpiniaceae
15.	*Catharanthus roseus* (L.) Don	Apocynaceae
16.	*Cleistanthus collinus* (Roxb.) Benth.ex-.Hook.f.	Euphorbiaceae
17.	*Cryptostegia grandiflora* Roxb. ex. R.Br.	Apocynaceae
18.	*Cuscuta reflexa* Roxb.	Cuscutaceae
19.	*Datura metel* L.	Solanaceae

20.	*Datura stramonium* L.	Solanaceae
21.	*Dioscorea bulbifera* L.	Dioscoreaceae
22.	*Euphorbia antiquorum* L.	Euphorbiaceae
23.	*Euphorbia cyathophora* L.	Euphorbiaceae
24.	*Euphorbia hirta* L.	Euphorbiaceae
25.	*Euphorbia milii* L.	Euphorbiaceae
26.	*Euphorbia neriifolia* L.	Euphorbiaceae
27.	*Euphorbia nivulia* Buch-Ham.	Euphorbiaceae
28.	*Euphorbia pulcherrima* Willd.	Euphorbiaceae
29.	*Euphorbia tirucalli* L.	Euphorbiaceae
30.	*Excoecarica agallocha* L.	Euphorbiaceae
31.	*Gloriosa superba* L.	Colchicaceae
32.	*Jatropha curcas* L.	Euphorbiaceae
33.	*Jatropha gossypifolia* L.	Euphorbiaceae
34.	*Lantana camara* L.	Verbenaceae
35.	*Melia azedarach* L.	Meliaceae
36.	*Momordica charantia* L.	Cucurbitaceae
37.	*Moringa oleifera* Lam.	Moringaceae
38.	*Mucuna pruriens* (Linn) DC.	Fabaceae
39.	*Nerium oleander* L.	Apocynaceae
40.	*Nicotiana tabacum* L.	Solanaceae
41.	*Oxalis corniculata* L.	Oxalidaceae
42.	*Parthenium hysterophors* L.	Asteraceae
43.	*Pedilanthus tithymaloides* (L.) Poit.	Euphorbiaceae
44.	*Plumbago zeylanica* L.	Plumbaginaceae
45.	*Plumeria rubra* L.	Apocynaceae
46.	*Punica granatum* L.	Punicaceae
47.	*Rauvolfia serpentina* (L.) Benth. ex. Kurz.	Apocynaceae
48.	*Ricinus communis* L.	Euphorbiaceae

49.	*Solanum nigrum* L.	Solanaceae
50.	*Solanum virginianum* L.	Solanaceae
51.	*Strychnos nux-vomica* L.	Loganiaceae
52.	*Urginea indica* (Roxb.) Kunth.	Liliaceae

Contents

MEDICINAL AND POISONOUS PLANTS OF INDIA

Introduction

Literally thousands of plants contain various quantities of poisonous substances. Poisonous plants are a little group of plants that yield phytochemical constituents, which exert harmful causes or effect death either presently or by purpose of cumulative activity of the toxic substances due to presence of known or unknown phytochemical principles in it and not by mechanical activity (Chopra *et al.,* 1949). The poisonous quality of complete plant or any plant part may be due to production of phytotoxic substances namely, glycosides, phenolic toxicants, resins, tannins, saponins, proteins, amino acids, amines, mycotoxins, alkaloids, carbohydrates, chelating poisons, metals, ketones, essential oil, picrotoxins, toxalbumins, etc. Several of these are detrimental to man and animal life, at least under particular conditions.

There are some poisonous plants that grow in India. As people of India are not able to identify which plants are poisonous, women and children are prone to be victimized by eating poisonous plants accidently. Sometimes single plant species possesses both poisonous and therapeutic value. The poisonous plants of India have been described by many authors (Chopra *et al.,* 1984; Jain, 1999; Katewa *et al.,* 2008; Jangid and Sharma, 2011). The word "poisonous" means that the plant or plant part will effect some type of troubling cause and that produce may be a extensive extent of disorders. Some plants or part of plant may exhibit a mild poisonous effect while others may even lead to death.

Toxins are molecules that are noxious to living organisms. It is a truth that virtually any essence can be hurtful at extreme sufficient concentrations - as Paracelsus (1943-1951) the father of toxicology said in the 16th century, "the dose makes the toxin". Toxins accommodate both originally created compounds and chemicals produced by humans. Genuine poisons are produced by species of plants, fungi, bacteria, protists and animals. Poisonous plants are those which effect dangerous problems or even cause death, if a tiny quantity of its leaves, stem, seeds, fruits and roots are ingested (Greval, 1953). Several other plants are usually secure but they may become toxic if preparative from them are taken in excess in potent doses or for a long period of time as suggested by Qureshi *et al.,* 2001.

Several plants are poisonous to varying degrees that an enumeration would be useless. Numerous plants used for their psychological effects are poisonous if utilized in great quantities. It is complicated to identify exactly how humans discovered which plants were or were not toxic and the quantities that could be relatively safe for ingestion.

Several plants contain a great number of biologically active phytochemicals which are excessively helpful for curing several human and animal ailments. But absolutely a few flowering plants / herbs / shrubs or trees look innocent but cause dangerous sickness or death of human beings and animals. These plants which are detrimental to human or livestock are known as poisonous plants. Information on poisonous plants is as significant as medicinal plants because some of them are also utilized in drug preparation. It is very complicated to trace a clear border line between medicinal and poisonous plants because most of these plants condition for both the division. Poisonous / toxic plants are the elements of ethnomedicine. People not only utilize medicinal plants but also poisonous plants having some other significance in various uses. The interrelationship of medicinal and poisonous properties of plant is significant as medicinal effectiveness occurs at a lesser quantity whereas overdosing can cause poisoning. These have poisonous cause on contact, inhalation or by absorption or ingestion. However, noxious plants may include active phytochemical constituents with serviceable biological properties (Mchaw and Eloff, 2005).

Some of the plant toxins include *Strychnos nux-vomica, Nerium oleander, Datura metel* and gastro-intestinal irritants namely, *Ricinus communis, Calotropis gigantea, Croton tiglium,* etc. (Qureshi *et al.,* 2001). Poisonous plants of India have been reported by few workers (Viswanathan and Joshi, 1983; Ballantyne *et al.,* 1995; Singh *et al.,* 1999; Alagesaboopathi, 2012; Pasayat *et al.,* 2013).

Several plants grown in forest have poisonous qualities. Poisonous plants are plants, which as an entire or part thereof under all or particular conditions and in a method and in total likely to be taken or brought into contact with an organism will exert harmful causes or effects death either suddenly or by reason of cumulative performance of the poisonous effects due to presence of known or unknown biochemical essences in it and not by mechanical activity (Chopra *et al.,* 1949). People utilize not only the medicinal plants but also the poisonous plants having several other benefits in various application knowingly or unknowingly. Because individual plant contains lots of phytochemical constituents which do not indicate uniformity in activity, particularly children are prone to be victimized by eating poisonous plants accidentally. The poisonous plant parts may be leaves, root, stem, seeds, tubers, root bark, stem bark, fruits, latex, flowers, seed shell, green berry, pods hairs or even entire plant (Chopra, *et al.,* 1949; Chopra *et al.,* 1965; Katewa *et al.,* 2008; Rakhi Gupta, 2010; Jangid and Sharma, 2011; Alagesaboopathi, 2012; Pasayat *et al.,* 2013).

Poisonous plants are a little group of plants that exhibit phytochemical constituents, which exert directly or indirectly toxic activities and intervene in the metabolism of human beings and animals. These plants are found all around us. In the residence, various potted plants and floral decorations are really poisonous. Others may be harmful simply because of allergies.

Many of us are not known with these familiar poisonous plants that effect skin irritations. We do not recognize popular ornamental plants in the landscape that may effect inner poisoning when ingested. Underage children, adults or pets sometimes eat the fruit or leaves of ornamental plants in the landscape which are poisonous. Many plants may be only mildly toxic and may cause stomach ache or mild irritation of the throat and mouth when ingested. There are also a number of changeables that decide how dangerous the poisoning indications may be such as the age, weight and health position of a person in connection to the amount of the plant ingested as well as the form that the plant was in at the time of ingestion, which include cooked versus raw, ripe fruit versus unripe fruit, etc.

The poisonous plants cause toxicity due to presence of organic compounds, which interrupt with human metabolic mode or enzymatic method causing toxicity. Aminoacids, phenolic toxicants, alkaloids, glycosides, alcohols, ketones, carbohydrates, lipids, metals, proteins, mycotoxins, chelating poisons are the essences or chemicals which are answerable for poisonous potentialities of plants. Every part of the individual poisonous plant may not accommodate the poisonous ingredients as the distribution of poisonous essences is irregular. Sometimes individual plant species exhibit both poisonous and medicinal value. The possession of poisonous ingredients gave particular plants a scanty benefit in the struggle for existence (Rakhi Gupta *et al.*, 2010).

Investigations on poisonous activities of plants in the wild were made by several researchers (Watt and Breyer-Brandwijk, 1962; Chopra *et al.*, 1984; Cheze *et al.*, 2000; Furler *et al.*, 2000; Agra *et al.*, 2007; Katewa *et al.*, 2008; Rakhi Gupta *et al.*, 2010; Jangid and Sharma, 2011; Alagesaboopathi, 2012; Pasayat, 2013).

India is endowed with a rich wealth of medicinal plants which have been a valuable source of natural products for maintaining human health. Numerous life threatening side effects also developed on usage of some synthetic medicines in the treatment of certain ailments. Herbal medicines are also the treatment options which are available and affordable to the rural populace depending on traditional medicines for their primary healthcare necessities (Lawal *et al.*, 2013). Large number of these medicinal plants are used in various formulations for the treatment of several diseases caused by microbes. According to World Health Organization (WHO), medicinal plants would be the source in obtaining a variety of drugs. Several societies across the world have shown great interest in curing ailments using plants / plant-based drugs. Microbes are closely associated with the health and welfare of human beings. Some are beneficial and some are detrimental. As preventive and curative measures, plants and their products are used in the treatment of infections since several centuries ago. WHO estimated that 80 percentage of the people worldwide rely on plant-based medicines for their primary healthcare needs (Fransworth, 1994; Alagesaboopathi, 2011) and India happens to be the largest user of traditional medical treatment, using 7000 plant species.

The increasing failure of chemotherapies and antibiotic resistance exhibited by pathogenic microbial infectious agent have led to the screening of various medicinal plants for their potential antimicrobial activity (Ritch-Krc *et al.*, 1996; Martins, *et al.*, 2001; Alagesaboopathi, 2011). Antibacterial properties of various plants parts such as rhizomes, roots, stem, leaves, seeds and fruits have been well documented for some of the medicinal plants for the past two decades (Leven, *et al.*, 1979). Antibiotic principles are distributed widely among angiospermic plants. A variety of compounds are accumulated in plant parts accounting for their constitutive antimicrobial properties. Herbal medicine represents one of the most important fields of traditional medicine all over the world. Many plants in the world are being tested for antimicrobial activities and the results derived from these scientific studies have aided in the validation of traditional uses of these plants (Edewor, *et al.*, 2012). The world is lush with naturally grown medicinal plants. In India, 500 medicinal plant species are used to control pathogenic bacteria (Bhuvaneshwari *et al.*, 2006). Plants have been used as traditional medicine since time immemorial to control bacterial, viral and fungal diseases.

Medicinal plants are now more focused than ever because they have the capability of producing many benefits to society indeed to mankind, especially in the line of medicine and pharmacological (Hussain *et al.*, 2011a). Plant-based drugs have been in use against various diseases since time immemorial (Hussain *et al.*, 2011b). Any parts of plant: rhizome, root, stem, leaves, flowers, seeds and fruits etc. which have one or more of its organs constituents that can be utilized for therapeutic purposes, are called medicinal plants (Hussain *et al.*, 2011c). It is a fact that the 25% of all medical prescriptions are based on substances derived from plants or plant-derived synthetic analogues (Ullah *et al.*, 2010). There is a great contribution of medicinal plants in the human health for the treatment of different ailments. Plants are the main source of anti-infective agents like emetine, quinine and berberine that are highly effective instruments in the fight against microbial infections. Phytoremedies have also shown great promise in the treatment of intractable infectious diseases, including opportunistic AIDS infections (Loiy *et al.*, 2011). The phytochemical constituents and medicinal properties of most of the medicinal plants were recorded in the last few decades by a number of workers (Nudrat *et al.*, 2005; Riazullah *et al.*, 2012; Ilango *et al.*, 2012). These medicinal plants are subjected to several processes and then administrated to the patients. The survey and documentation of medicinally important plants in each and every place is very much important for easy identification of local traditional healers, conservation and sustainable utilization. Antibacterial and antifungal properties of medicinal plants parts such as leaf stem and root have been well noted for some of the medicinal plants for the past two decades. Medicinal plants and their essences are wealth of antibacterial compounds that can fight against bacterial ailments (Meera *et al.*, 1999).

Indian medicinal plants and their products are used to control diverse disease such as catarrh, bronchitis, pneumonia, ulcers and diarrhoea. Researchers are increasingly turning their attention to folk medicine looking for new leads to develop better drugs against cancer, as well as viral and microbial infections (Galal *et al.*, 1991; Hoffimann *et al.*, 1993). Although hundreds of plant species have been tested for antimicrobial properties, the vast majority have not yet been adequately evaluated (Balandrin *et al.*, 1985). In every developing country it is necessary that the documentation of medicinal plants be treated as a matter of extreme urgency.

The search for plants with antimicrobial activity has gained increasing importance in modern years due to growing worldwide concern about the alarming increase in the rate of infection by antibiotic-resistant microorganism (Salvat *et al.,* 2004). Medicinal plants would be the best source to obtain a variety of drugs (Santos *et al.,* 1995). As preventive and curative measures, plants and their products are used in the treatment of infections since many centuries ago.

In addition to the alarming increase in the incidence of modern and re-emerging infectious diseases, one major health concern is the resistance to existing antibiotics (Agbarfor *et al.,* 2011). Furthermore, novel antibiotics in the drug, development pipeline that offers significant benefits over existing drugs is lacking (Butler *et al.,* 2011). It is largely known that plants possess healing properties (Imaga, 2010). Such properties can be partly attributed to the diverse array of secondary metabolites (i.e., terpenes, alkaloids, phenolic compounds and cyanogenic glycosides) which are known to be essential for plants defense against microbial attack (Cowan, 1999; Dixon, 2001; Oseni *et al.,* 2011). Treatment of common infections with medicinal plant has been familiar in developing countries due to its cheaper cost and claims for both its effectiveness and lesser side effects over synthetic drug (Menghani *et al.,* 2011). A diverse range of compounds that offer potentials for the treatment of chronic and infectious disease can be found most especially in traditional medicinal plants (Duraipandiyan *et al.,* 2006).

India is known as the botanical garden of the world. Out of the complete 4,22,000 flowering plants documented from the world, more than 50,000 are utilized for medicinal applications (Govaerts, 2001). In India, more than 43 percentage of the whole flowering plants are noted to be of medicinal significance (Pushpangandan, 1995). Utilization of plants for medicinal purposes in India has been reported long back in ancient literature (Charak, 1996). The identification and documentation of plants of ethnomedicinal significance in various cultures have long been a dynamic area of investigation and has been connected with many objectives.

Utilization of medicinal plants as a source of medicine to treat several ailments is as old as humankind itself. Even to the present day, medicinal plants are usable as inexpensive and available source of medicine for most of developing and also developed countries. The World Health Organization (WHO) has been continuously emphasizing the utilization of herbal and traditional medicines. The organization has also evaluated that about 80 percentage of the population living in the developing countries rely on traditional drug for their healthcare claims (WHO, 2002).

The utilization of plants as drug is widespread throughout the world. People of various areas of the world have been using medicinal plants for treatment of several diseases for thousands of years (Hill, 1989). With the advent of recent or allopathic medication, traditional medicinal usages are refused to some extent. However, in current years, traditional or herbal drug has been recognized from both patients and doctors. About 64 percentage of the whole worldwide population still remains dependent on traditional medicine for their healthcare necessities (Cotto, 1996).

Research of Medicinal and Poisonous Plants

The inhabitants are well perceptive of the medicinal and poisonous potentialities of plants growing in and around their surroundings. The knowledge has been passed on from generation to generation as a guarded secret. Each tribe has its main medicine-man and has its main set of medications. Efforts were made to collect data from the area and an inventory has been prepared. For identification of plants, various related floras, monographs and other works were consulted at the Department of Botany, Government Arts College (Autonomous), Salem-7, Tamilnadu. An alphabetical list of species with scientific name, vernacular name, botanical description, distribution, propagation, plant parts used, phytochemical constituents, medicinal uses, toxic constituents, poisonous parts and poisonous symptoms has been prepared. Medicinal worthiness of plants have been ascertained in consultation with Maheswari 2000; Pandikumar *et al.,* 2007; Karuppusamy, 2007; Ganesan, 2008; Alagesaboopathi, 2009, 2011; Rajendran and Manian, 2011; Arunachalam and Parimelazhagan, 2011; Jeyaprakash *et al.,* 2011; David and Sudarsanam, 2011; Chew *et al.,* 2012; Ayyanar, 2013; Vaidyanathan *et al.,* 2014; Maria Francis Jeffrey Bose *et al.,* 2014; Salai Senthilkumar *et al.,* 2014; Alagesaboopathi, 2014 and Mukeshkumar *et al.,*

2014. Poisonous plants have been ascertained in reports by Katewa *et al.*, 2008; Rakhi *et al.*, 2010; Jangid and Sharma, 2011; Alagesaboopathi, 2012; Pasayat *et al.*, 2013; Adediwura *et al.*, 2014; Poonam Agarwal, 2014 and Bhatia *et al.*, 2014.

The familiar medicinal uses and poisonous symptoms were known from literature. Tribals, village dwellers, rural populace, the herbal medicine practitioner and other traditional healers were interviewed for recording the unique information about medicinal values of various plant species with their vernacular names. Medicinal plants are a vital principle of synthetic and herbal medicines. The recent pharmaceutical industry also requires an enormous content of authentic plants for the produce of their medicines. Extraction of active properties and manufacture of medicine formulations require sophisticated technology and leading investment. Medicinal plants are considered to be a chemical factory, comprising of varied phytochemical compounds such as flavonoids, tannins, phenolic compounds, triterpenoids, saponins, terpenoids, steroids, sterols, resins, glycosides, oils, oleoresins, sesquiterpene lactones, alkaloids etc. Today there is growing attention in phytochemical competition of plant-based drugs. Various phytochemical constituents have been isolated and studied for p harmacological, chemical and clinical activities. Now-a-days, based on the primitive information in folk remedies, there is an increasing demand for the production of healthcare medicines and cosmetic fields from plant derivation.

The total number of medicinal and poisonous plants are 52 (Table 1), out of which the greatest number of medicinal and poisonous plants are under the family Euphorbiaceae, Fabaceae, Solanaceae, Apocynaceae, followed by Asclepiadaceae, Asteraceae, Verbenaceae, Colchicaceae, Oxalidaceae, Cuscutaceae and Caricaceae.

Abrus Precatorius L.

Family: Fabaceae

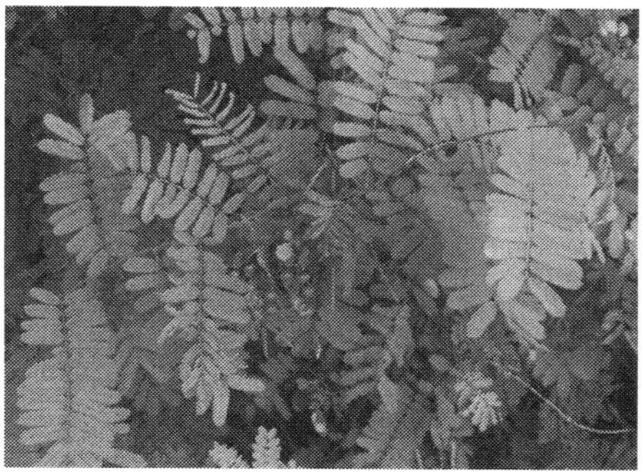

Vernacular Names : *Gunja* (Sanskrit), *Rati, Gunchi* (Hindi), *Kunch, Koonch* (Bengali), *Gumchi, Chanothi* (Gujarati), *Shangir* (Kashmiri), *Gurugunji* (Kannada), *Kunni, Gundumani* (Malayalam), *Mulati* (Punjabi), *Gundumani, Kunthamani* (Tamil), *Guruvenda* (Telugu), *Gunja, Gunchi* (Marathi), *Raturmani* (Assam).

Botanical Description: A beautiful, much-branched, slender, perennial, deciduous, woody, prickly twining or smooth, textured, brown. Leaves are stipulate, pinnately compound, leaflets 7-24 pairs, 0.6-2.5 x 0.4-1.2 cm, turgid, oblong, obtuse at both ends, appressed hairy. Flowers in axillary racemes, shorter than leaves, pink or pinkish-white. Calyx-lobes short, appressed hairy. Pods 1.6-5.1x0.8-1.6 cm, turgid, oblong, appressed hairy, with a sharp deflexed beak, silky-textured, 3 to 6 seeded. Seeds elliptic to sub-globose, *ca* 0.5 cm in diam; smooth, glossy, shinning red with black blotch around the hilum.

Flowering and Fruiting: August–January.

Distribution: Throughout India, Sri Lanka, Thailand, Philippine Islands, South China, tropical Africa and the West Indies.

Propagation: By seeds

Parts Used: Leaves, roots and seeds

Phytochemical Constituents: Abricin, abrin, abrasine, abraline, abrine, abrusgenic acid, abruslactone, abrussic-acid, anthocyanins, abrusgenic-acid-methyl ester, choline, campesterol, glycyrrhizin, hypaphorine, gallic acid, pectin, pentosan-s N, n-dimethyl-tryptophan, N-n-dimethyl-tryptophan-metho-cation-methyl ester, P-coumaroylgalloyl-glulodelphinidin, hypaphorine, picatorine.

Medicinal Uses: The seeds are antimicrobial, cytotoxic, diuretic, emetic, antitumor, aphrodisiac, anodyne, febrifuge, laxative, purgative, sedative, vermifuge, antidote, expectorant, emollient, hemostat, and used in several diseases to cure snake bite, boil, cancer, cold, cough, diarrhoea, fever, gonorrhea, jaundice, headache, malaria, rheumatism, ophthalmia and night-blindness. The seeds are also used to manage diabetes and chronic nephritis. The leaves are used for their anti-suppurative properties, tetanus, and to prevent rabies. Paste of roots is administered to cure abdominal pains and tumors. The paste with fresh rhizome of *Curcuma longa* is externally applied on wounds.

Poisonous Parts: Seeds

Toxic Constituents: Abrine, abrin and abrasine.

Poisonous Symptoms: Seeds are poisonous and causes vomiting, diarrhoea, nausea, shock, convulsions, as well as induce direct toxicity on the kidneys, cardiac poison, paralysis, gastroenteritis with purging and temperature fluctuation followed by death. Seeds are eaten by livestock, which causes vomiting, severe diarrhoea and weakness. The seed extract can cause eye injury.

Abrus Precatorius L. (Black seed variety)

Family: Fabaceae

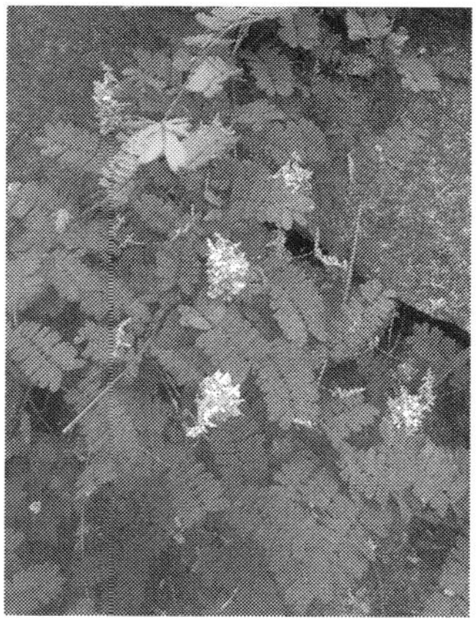

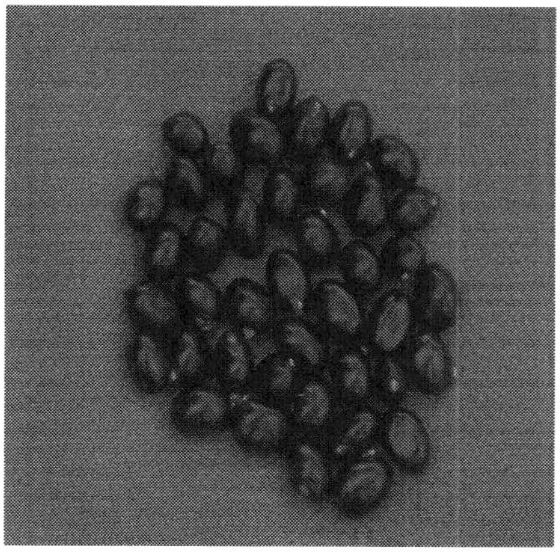

Seeds

Vernacular Names: *Black Gundumani* (Tamil)

Botanical Description: A beautiful, much-branched, slender, perennial, deciduous, woody, prickly twining or smooth, textured, brown. Leaves are stipulate, pinnately compound, leaflets 7-24 pairs,

0.6-2.5 x 0.4-1.2 cm, turgid, oblong, obtuse at both ends, appressed hairy. Flowers in axillary racemes, shorter than leaves, pink or pinkish-white. Calyx-lobes short, appressed hairy. Pods 1.6-5.1x0.8-1.6 cm, turgid, oblong, appressed hairy, with a sharp deflexed beak, silky-textured, 3 to 6 seeded. Seeds elliptic to sub-globose, *ca* 0.5 cm in diam; smooth, glossy, shinning red with black blotch around the hilum.

Flowering and Fruiting: September–December

Distribution: Tamilnadu, particularly in Eastern Ghats

Propagation: By seeds

Parts Used: Roots, leaves and seeds

Phytochemical Constituents: Abricin, abrin, abrasine, abraline, abrine, abrusgenic acid, abruslactone, abrussic-acid, anthocyanins, abrusgenic-acid-methyl ester, choline, campesterol, glycyrrhizin, hypaphorine, gallic acid, pectin, pentosan-s N, n-dimethyl-tryptophan, N-n-dimethyl-tryptophan-metho-cation-methyl ester, P-coumaroylgalloyl-glulodelphinidin, hypaphorine, picatorine.

Medicinal Uses: The seeds are used in treating jaundice, arthritis, skin diseases, purgative, snake bite, scorpion sting and leucoderma. The aerial parts decoction is also used for treating certain infections like diarrhoea, leucorrhoea, gonorrhea and dysentery. Root juice is useful for ulcer, diarrhoea and abdominal pains.

Poisonous Parts: Seeds.

Toxic Constituents: Abrine, abrin and abrasine

Poisonous Symptoms: Intake of seeds causes paralysis, vomiting, nausea, diarrhoea, extreme fever and lastly death. Consumption of seeds by livestock results in salivation, shivering, severe diarrhoea, abortion in pregnant livestock and even death.

Abrus Precatorius L. (Red seed variety)

Family: Fabaceae

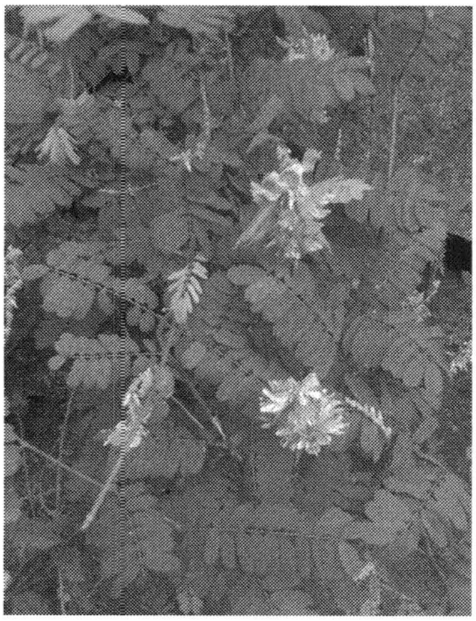

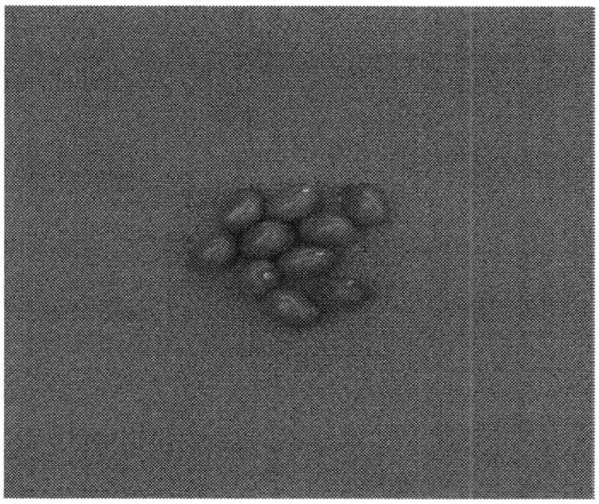

Seeds

Vernacular Names: *Red Gundumani* (Tamil)

Botanical Description: A beautiful, much-branched, slender, perennial, deciduous, woody, prickly twining or smooth, textured, brown. Leaves stipulate, pinnately compound, leaflets 7-24 pairs,

0.6-2.5x0.4-1.2 cm, turgid, oblong, obtuse at both ends, appressed hairy. Flowers in axillary racemes, shorter than leaves, pink or pinkish-white. Calyx-lobes short, appressed hairy. Pods 1.6-5.1x0.8-1.6 cm, turgid, oblong, appressed hairy, with a sharp deflexed beak, silky-textured, 3 to 6 seeded. Seeds elliptic to sub-globose, *ca* 0.5 cm in diam; smooth, glossy, shinning red with black blotch around the hilum.

Flowering and Fruiting: August - January

Distribution: Tamilnadu, particularly in Salem, Dharmapuri and Namakkal districts.

Propagation: By seeds

Parts Used: Whole plant

Phytochemical Constituents: Abricin, abrin, abrasine, abraline, abrine, abrusgenic acid, abruslactone, abrussic-acid, anthocyanins, abrusgenic-acid-methyl ester, choline, campesterol, glycyrrhizin, hypaphorine, gallic acid, pectin, pentosan-s N, n-dimethyl-tryptophan, N-n-dimethyl-tryptophan-metho-cation-methyl ester, P-coumaroylgalloyl- glulodelphinidin, hypaphorine, picatorine.

Medicinal Uses: The whole plant powder mixed with Cow's milk is given orally for cough, ulcer, fever and asthma. Seed paste is applied externally for snake bite, scorpion sting, ulcers, inflammatory conditions, scabies and healing of wounds.

Poisonous Parts: Seeds

Toxic Constituents: Abrine, abrin and abrasine

Poisonous Symptoms: Consumption of seeds causes diarrhoea, vomiting, nausea, throat pain and inflammation in eyes. Seeds when eaten by animals cause severe diarrhoea, nasal discharge, weakness and even death.

Abrus Precatorius L. (White seed variety)

Family: Fabaceae

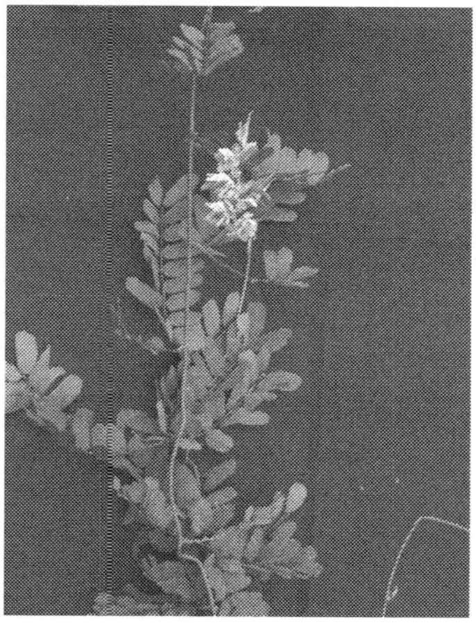

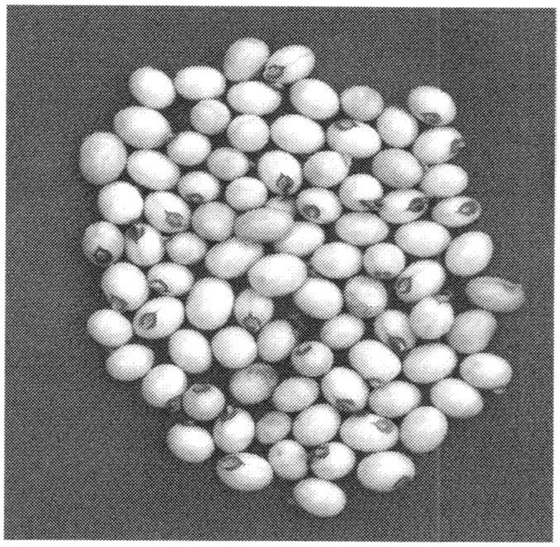

Vernacular Names: *Indian Liquorice* (English), *White kundumani* (Tamil), *Kumi* (Malayalam), *Rektika, Gunja* (Sanskrit), *Gunchi, Ratti* (Hindi), *Gulganji* (Kannada).

Botanical Description: A climbing, woody, vine grows up to 4-6 m height, leaves alternate, compound, feather-like, with small oblong leaflets. Petals rose to pink, stamens 9, flowers are many and appear in the leaf axils along the stems. 3-10 cm long, red to purple or white fruit legume, 4 cm long, seeds, ovoid, ellipsoid, hard textured and of smooth surface, compressed, white colour flowers produce white coloured seeds, 5.4-6.1 mm in length and 2.9-4.3 mm in width. Seeds white with a black spot.

Flowering and Fruiting: August–December

Distribution: Throughout India, particularly in Tamilnadu, Madhya Pradesh, Uttar Pradesh, Andhra Pradesh.

Propagation: By seeds

Parts Used: Roots, leaves and seeds

Phytochemical Constituents: The seeds contain flavonoids, steroids, alkaloids, trite penoids, saponins, gums and mucilages, tannins, phenolic compounds, protein and amino acids, fixed oils and fats.

Medicinal Uses: The seeds are useful in treating eye disease, jaundice, pain, arthritis, leucoderma and poisonous bite. Seed paste is used as antiseptic, abortifacient, antitubercular, antidiabetic, antidysentric, and also useful for treating paralysis, skin diseases, ulcer, inflammation and eye disorders. The leaves are useful in tetanus and anti-suppurative activities. A paste of the seed is given in purgative, nervous diseases, gonorrhoea, hair loss and delivery pain. It is also useful for cytotoxicity, anti-inflammatory, antibacterial, snake bite, diabetes, wound healing, cancer, fever ulcer, asthma, leprosy, tumor and tubercular glands. The leaves and roots are diuretic, alexeteric, astringent, anthelmintic and sweet. They are useful in treatment of inflammation, cough, strangury, pectroalgia and pharyngodynia. The seeds are purgative, astringent, toxic, abortifacient, bitter, acrid, trichogenous and aphrodisiac. Seeds paste is applied on affected part in skin ailments, asthma, paralysis, wounds, stomatitis, fever, alopecia, sciatica, stiffness of shoulder joints, tubercular glands and hyperdipsia.

Poisonous Parts: Seeds

Toxic Constituents: Abrine, abrin and abrasine.

Poisonous Symptoms: Intake of seeds causes cardiac poison, paralysis, vomiting, high fever, inflammation in eyes and temperature fluctuation followed by death. Seeds along with other plant parts intake by animals result in shivering, salivation, acute diarrhoea and even death.

Abrus Precatorius L. (Yellow seed variety)

Family: Fabaceae

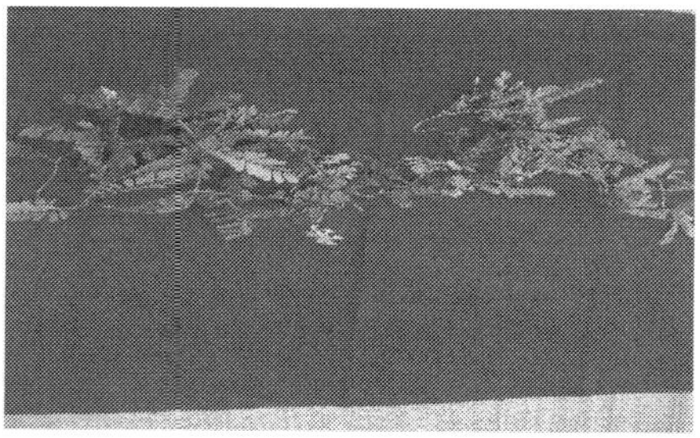

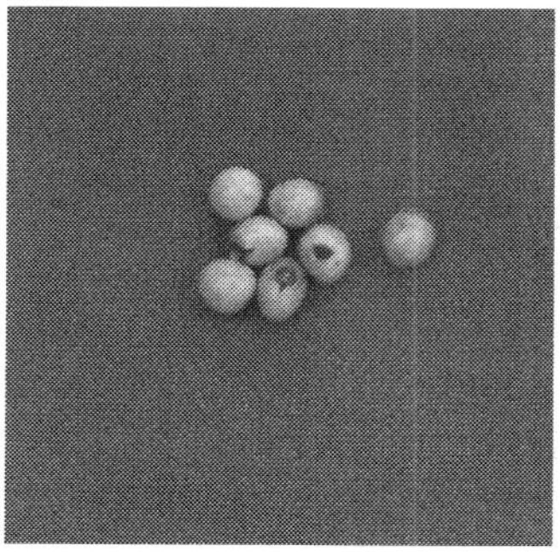

Seeds

Vernacular Names: *Yellow Gundumani* (Tamil)

Botanical Description: A beautiful, much-branched, slender, perennial, deciduous, woody, prickly twining or smooth, textured, brown. Leaves stipulate, pinnately compound, leaflets 7-24 pairs, 0.6-2.5x0.4-1.2 cm, turgid, oblong, obtuse at both ends, appressed hairy. Flowers in axillary racemes, shorter than leaves, pink or pinkish-white. Calyx-lobes short, appressed hairy. Pods 1.6-5.1x0.8-1.6 cm, turgid, oblong, appressed hairy, with a sharp deflexed beak, silky-textured, 3 to 6 seeded. Seeds elliptic to sub-globose, *ca* 0.5 cm in diam; smooth, glossy, shining red with black blotch around the hilum.

Flowering and Fruiting: August–December

Distribution: Tamilnadu, particularly in Eastern Ghats

Propagation: By seeds

Parts Used: Leaves, roots and seeds

Phytochemical Constituents: Abricin, abrin, abrasine, abraline, abrine, abrusgenic acid, abruslactone, abrussic-acid, anthocyanins, abrusgenic-acid-methyl ester, choline, campesterol, glycyrrhizin, hypaphorine, gallic acid, pectin, pentosan-s N, n-dimethyl-tryptophan, N-n-dimethyl-tryptophan-metho cation-methyl ester, P-coumaroylgalloyl-glulodelphinidin, hypaphorine, picatorine.

Medicinal Uses: The seeds are used in snake bite, scorpion sting, skin ailments, eye troubles, diabetes,

	arthritis and inflammation. Root paste mixed with coconut oil is applied to treat skin diseases. Fresh decoction of the leaves is anthelmintic, and cures fever, jaundice, ulcer and diarrhoea.
Poisonous Parts:	Seeds
Toxic Constituents:	Abrine, abrin and abrasine
Poisonous Symptoms:	Seeds are poisonous and causes vomiting, high fever, inability to stand, gastroenteritis with purging, weakness, trembling of hands and lastly death. Intake of seeds by animals results in severe diarrhoea, vomiting and weakness.

Alangium Salvifolium (L.f.) Wangerin.

Family : Alangiaceae

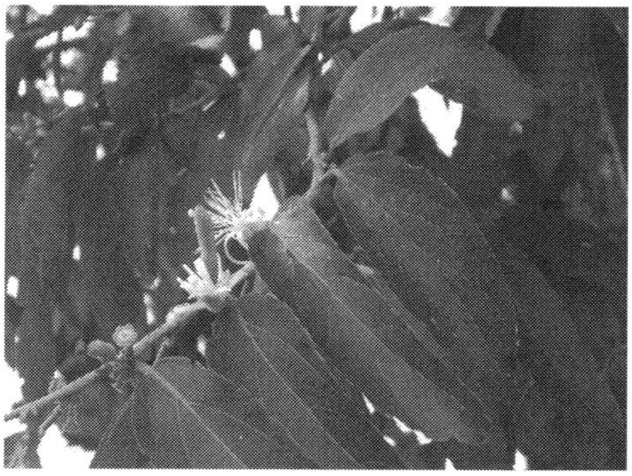

Vernacular Names: *Sage leaved Alangium* (English), *Alangimaram, Alangi* (Tamil), *Akola* (Hindi), *Ankol* (Sanskrit), *Ankol* (Gujarati), *Ankol* (Marathi), *Ankod, Dhala Ankor* (Bengali), *Ankule, Ankolmara* (Kannada), *Ankolam, Urgu* (Telugu), *Ankolam* (Malayalam).

Botanical Description: A small, thorny deciduous tree / shrub which grows up to a height of 5-30 meters with more or less pinescent branches. Bark yellowish. Leaves alternate, elliptical and leaves 7.4-15.1 cm long, narrowly oblong or ovate-lanceolate, glabrous. Usually unequal at the base; flowers-yellowish, white, fragrant in axillary fascides, fruits small, nearly globular, purplish-red when ripe, 1-2 seeded, 1.2 cm in length, 1-2 seeded berries crowned by the calyx-limb.

Flowering and Fruiting: February - July.

Distribution: Throughout the hotter parts of India, Sri Lanka and Southern and Eastern Asia, Philippines and tropical Australia.

Propagation: By seeds

Parts Used: Fruits, roots and leaves

Phytochemical Constituents: The plants contain alkaloids, cephaeline, psychotrine, marcking, ankorine, a and b-alangine, alangicin, marckindine, tubulosin, emitine and lamarckinine. Root bark contains the emetine, cephaeline, psychotrine, alkaloids, alangine and also myricyl alcohol. Stem bark contains the alangine, akharkantine, alkaloids, lamarkine and akoline.

Medicinal Uses: The leaves are useful in treating hypertension and are a useful antidote for various poisons especially for rabies. The root is useful for treating rheumatism, inflammation, and possesses diuretic, astringent and antidote properties. The fruit is useful as laxative and carminative; it is used to treat haemorrhages and burning sensation. It can exhibit emetic, purgative, antipyretic, diaphoretic, anthelmintic, febrifuge effect, and can treat fever, piles, skin diseases, leprosy and syphilitic. The plant is used to cure arthritis and possess antioxidant and antimicrobial properties.

Poisonous Parts: Root bark

Toxic Constituents: Alkaloids

Poisonous Symptoms: Intake of root bark decoction in small doses depresses heart; in large doses produces unusual respiration and transient fall in blood pressure.

Annona Squamosa L.

Family: Annonaceae

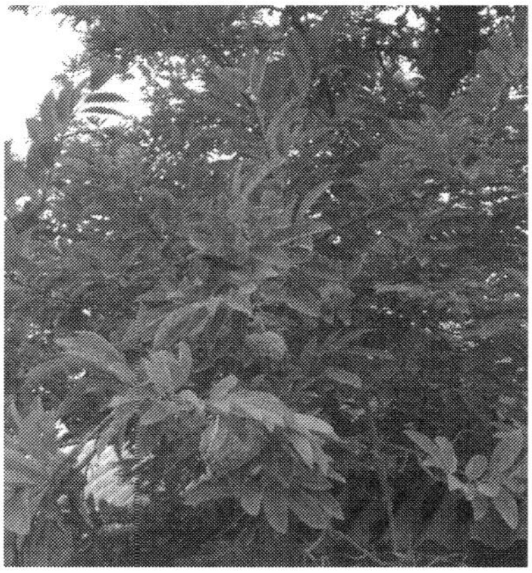

Vernacular Names : *Sugar apple, Custard apple, Sweet apres* (English), *Sharith, Sharifa, Sitaphal* (Hindi), *Sita*

Phalamn, Sitaphalam (Telugu), *Stiaphal* (Gujarati), *Ata* (Bengali), *Sitaphal* (Marathi), *Sitappalam, Seethapalam* (Tamil), *Sitaphalam* (Kannada), *Aathappazham, Seethapazham, Sirpha* (Malayalam)

Botanical Description: A woody semi-deciduous tree 3-8 m in height, with a wide, irregularly spreading branches, leaves eliptic, 5-18 x 3-7 cm, oblonglanceolate, or lanceolute, pale green on both surfaces and glabrate. Base short pointed or rounded, petioles 0.7 - 1.4 cm long, green, sparsely pubescent flowers 2-4 in a cluster, greenish-yellow, fragrant, on slender hairy stalks, produced singly, or in slight lateral clusters about 2.6m long. 2-4 flowers, sepals 3, triangular, pointed, green, hairy about 17mm long 3 outer petals 3, greenish yellow, oblong, thick, stamens very several, white, crowds, less than 17 mm long, ovary light green, styles white, fruit is round, heart shaped, conical or ovate, 6-12 cm diameter. The pulp is white, edible and sweetly aromatic. Seeds oblong, smooth and shiny, dark brown or blackish. 1.4-1.8 cm long many.

Flowering and Fruiting: July - November

Distribution: India, Thailand, West Indies, South America, Indonesia, Taiwan, Brazil, Malaysia, Pakistan, Sri Lanka, Philippines, China, Bangladesh, Cambodia, Vietnam, Argentina, Colombia, Australia, New Zealand and Uganda.

Propagation: By seeds

Parts Used: Leaves, bark, shoots, roots and fruits

Phytochemical Constituents:

The plant contains tannins, alkaloids, saponins, flavonoids, proteins, phenolic compounds, amino acids, glycosides, carbohydrates, phytosterols. The several phytochemicals isolated from root, stem and leaves of the plant including anonaine, coryeline, norcorydine, aprophine, glaucine, and isocorydine. The leaf contains camphene, carvone, camphor, car-3-ene, farnesol, eugenol, carphyllene, geraniol, hexacontanol, limonine, isocorydine, higemamine, linalool, acetate, borneol, a-pinene, b-pinene, rutin, menthone, methyl anthranilate, thymol, stigmasterol, glycosides, steroids, phenolic compounds and n-triacontanol.

Medicinal Uses:

The plant is considered serviceable for diabetes, cancer, cardiac disease and hyperthyroidism. The root is used to bring about drastic purgative activity. The plant also possesses antibacterial, antimicrobial, antioxidant, antihyperlipidemic, wound healing, diuretic, antidiabetic, anti-genotoxic agent, anti-head lice effect, hepatoprotective, cytotoxic, antitumour and insecticidal activity. It is used to perform larvicidal, anthelmintic activities, molluscicidal activity, mosquitocidal activity, antithyroidic activity, antiplasmodial activity, anti-platelet activity, vasorelaxant activity, and possess antiviral and antifertility properties. The plant is utilized to cure ulcer and inflammation.

A park decoction of this plant is useful to treat diarrhoea. Bark is used as potent vermifuge, astringent and antidysenteric agent. Root is used in the treatment of dysentery. Leaves are used to cure fainting spells. The leaves of the plant can act as anthelminitc, insecticide, styptic agent. The fruit is used as sedative, cooling agent, haematinic, stimulant, maturant tonic, and expectorant. They are utilized in curing anemia and burning sensation. The fruit is used in making ice creams and milk beverages.

Poisonous Parts: Seeds

Toxic Constituents: The seed oil contains annonastin and squamozin.

Poisonous Symptoms: Seed is poisonous; it is used as fish poison and insecticides.

Argemone Mexicana L.

Family: Papaveraceae

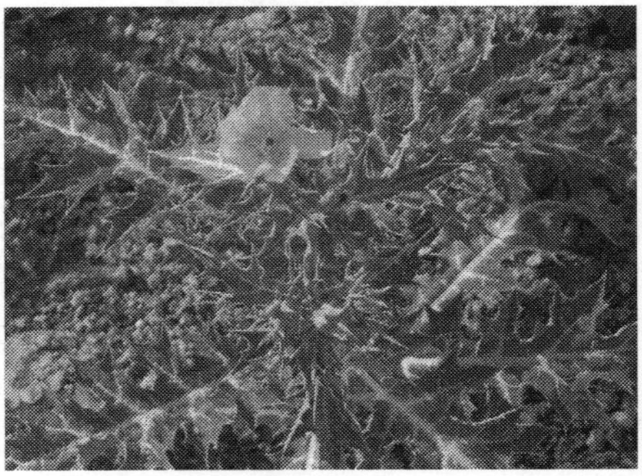

Vernacular Names: *Mexican prickly poppy* (English), *Brahmadandi, Pitopusha* (Sanskrit), *Ponnummattu* (Malayalam), *Satyanashi* (Hindi), *Kutiyotti, Ponnummuttai, Perammathandu* (Tamil), *Darudi* (Gujarati), *Brahmadandi cettu* (Telugu).

Botanical Description: A strong glabrous, branching annual herb with yellow juice and showy yellow flowers, the height of this plant varies between 65-95 cm, leaves simple, sessile, spiny, semi-amplexcaul, spinous. Stem clasping, oblong, sinuately pinnatified, spinous and viens are white, flowers are terminal, yellow and of 2.8 - 5.2 cm diameter. Fruits are capsule. Prickly and oblong ovoid. Seeds numerous, globose, netted and brownish black.

Flowering and Fruiting: October - March.

Distribution: Throughout India and Ethiopia.

Propagation: By seeds

Parts Used: Roots, leaves, seed, yellow juice, fruits, latex and flowers

Phytochemical Constituents: Berberine, argemexitin, 5,7-dihydroxychromone-7-neohesperidoside (I), eriodictyol, protopine, sarguinarine, chelerytherine, optisine, myristic, oleic, linoleic acids, palmitic, sanguinarine, dihydrosanguinarine, alkaloids, glycosides, saponins, tannins, flavonoids, carbohydrates and proteins.

Medicinal Uses: The whole plant is purgative, diuretic, destroys worms, leprosy, skin diseases, inflammations and bilious fevers. It can act as emetic, expectorant, demulcent, antitussive, sedative, warts, antispasmodic, analgesic and anthelmintic agent. The fresh yellow, milky, acrid sap contains protein-dissolving substances and has been used in the treatment of skin diseases, itches, cold sores, warts and cutaneous affections. The root is alternative and has been used in the treatment of chronic skin ailments. The flowers are expectorant and have been used in the treatment of coughs. The seed are emetics, laxative, expectorant, sedative, purgative and demulcent. The seed has also been used as an antidote to snake poisoning. It has been used in the treatment of skin diseases. The leaves are hepatoprotective and are also useful for treating skin ailments, ulcers, cough, wounds, leprosy, jaundice and malarial fever.

Poisonous Parts: All parts especially seeds

Toxic Constituents: Protopine, dihydro-sanguinarine, berberine and sanguinarine

Poisonous Symptoms: Fruits and seeds are narcotic and emetic causing vomiting, diarrhoea and headache. Fruits and seeds consumption in higher doses causes poisoning. The plant when eaten by livestock causes diarrhoea.

Calotropis Gigentia (L.) R.Br.

Family : Asclepiadaceae

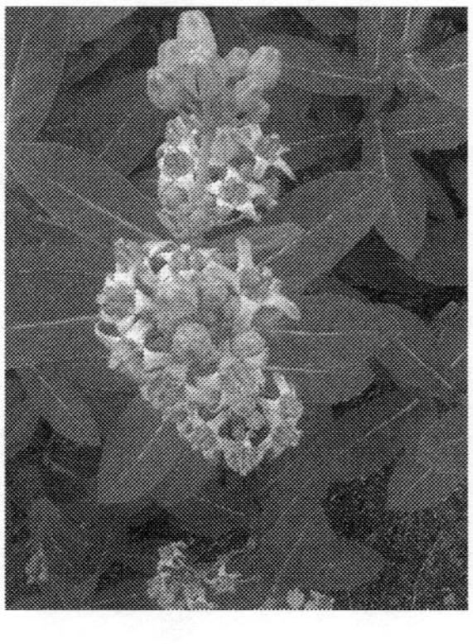

Vernacular Names: *Guint calotrope, Crown flower, Milkweed, Giant Milkweed, Madar* (English), *Madara, Akavan, Safed Aak, Arka, Mudar* (Hindi), *Erukku, Pellerukku* (Tamil), *Jilledu, Jilledipuuly, Nallajilledu, Mandaram* (Telugu), *Ak* (Punjabi), *Akado, Akad* (Gujarati), *Aakanda* (Bengali), *Akamadar, Rhi* (Marathi), *Angkot* (Manipuri), *Yerikku, Erikku, Dinesam* (Malayalam), *Alarka, Sadapuspa, Arki, Arka, Hrasvagnih* (Sanskrit).

Botanical Description: Large shrubs or a small tree up to 2.7 m height, stem rounded, leaves opposite-decussate, simple, sub sessile, blade-oblong, smaller in branchiets, elliptic-ovate to obovate, obtuse or apex, base cordate, lateral nerves 5-7 pairs. Flowers greenish-white or pale purple, complete, bisexual 3.1 cm across pedicels to 1-3 cm long, calyx, 5, polysepalous, 5 lobed, shortly united at the base. Corolla 5, Regular five lobed, gamopetalous, tube short, lobes ovate to oblong, recurved, stamens 5, gynandrous 1.1 cm long, fruit simple, fleshy inflated to 6.2 + 3.1 cm, ovoid seeds numerous, small, obovate, flat, compressed with silky white pappus.

Flowering and Fruiting: March to October

Distribution: Throughout India, French, Vietnam, Cambodia, Malaysia, Thailand, SriLanka, Indonesia, Philippines, China, Afghanistan, Iran, Jordan, Libya, Morocco, South Algeria, Egypt, Ethiopia, Eritrea, Iraq, Israel, Kenya, Mali, Nepal, Nigeria, Oman, Saudi Arabia, Uganda, Yemen, Sudan, Somalia, Brazil, Argentina, Bolivia, Chile, Cuba, Dominica, Colombia, Algeria, Jamaica, Panama, Paraguay, Peru, Mexico, Venezuela and Uruguay.

Propagation: By seeds.

Parts Used: Leaves, root bark and flowers.

Phytochemical Constituents: The plant yielded calotropin, calotoxin, gigantin, calactin, uscharin, alkaloids, phenols, tannins, flavonoids, steroids, saponins, terpenoids reducing sugar, resins. The latex contains calcium oxalate, cardio glycosides, volatile fatty acids Calotropain-FI, Calotropain FII, Calotropins DI and Calotropins DII. The plant is also contains phenolics, terpenes, cardenolides, protenases and nonprotein amino acid. The leaves yielded 15 beta-hydroxycardenolides, 16 alpha-hydroxy calactinic acid methyl ester and 19-Nor-and 18, 20-Epoxy-cardenolides. The flowers contain anhydrosophoradiol-3-acetate and Di-(2-ethylheyl) phthalate. The roots contain frusoside, calotrophenzofuranone, coroglancigenin, calotropises juiterpenol and calatropises terpenol. The root bark contains B-sitosterol, stigma sterol and gignaticine.

Medicinal Uses: The plant is used in treatment of epilepsy, leprosy, mental ailments, jaundice, skin disorders, elephantiasis, eczema, and can induce antimicrobial, cytotoxic, analgesic, antibacterial activity, anti-diarrhoeal activity, vermicidal activity, anti-candida activity, and antioxidant activity. Roots can induce cytotoxic activity, anti-pyretic activity, insecticidal activity, wound healing activity and pregnancy interceptive potentialities. Latex is utilized to manage antimicrobial property, dental problems, rare bite, gonococcal arthritis, swellings, wound healing activity, purgative properties and procoagulant activity. The stem possesses hepatoprotective properties. The leaves of *C.gigentia* are utilized in the remedy of swellings, paralysis and fevers. The leaves are also used for the curing of periodic fever, snake bites, vatha ailments, ulcers and intestinal worms. The flowers are used to treatment of catarrh, anorexia, asthma, fever, inflammations and helmintic infections. Root bark of the plant is used to manage cough, intestinal worms and cutaneous infections.

Poisonous Parts: Roots, leaves, fruit, latex and shoots.

Toxic Constituents: The latex contains many alkaloids namely, calotropin, calactin, calcilin, glycosides, catotoxin, gigantin, which are uscharin, caustic and regarded poisonous.

Poisonous Symptoms: Rapid dangerous corneal damage with painless immediate dimness of eyesight. In high doses the person undergoes uncontrollable convulsions until the lungs and heart fail from exhaustion. If the latex comes in contact with mucus or eyes it can cause burning sensation and excruciating pain. The flower juice is utilized to cause abortion for unwanted pregnancy. 25 ml of latex is given internally and causes female infant death. Both humans and livestock are affected by the latex as it is a potent irritant to skin. Accidental contact with eyes causes acute inflammation, along with redness. Leaves cause diarrhoea, drastic purgation and abortion in pregnant animals.

Calotropis Procera (Aiton) W.T. Aiton
Family: Asclepiadaceae

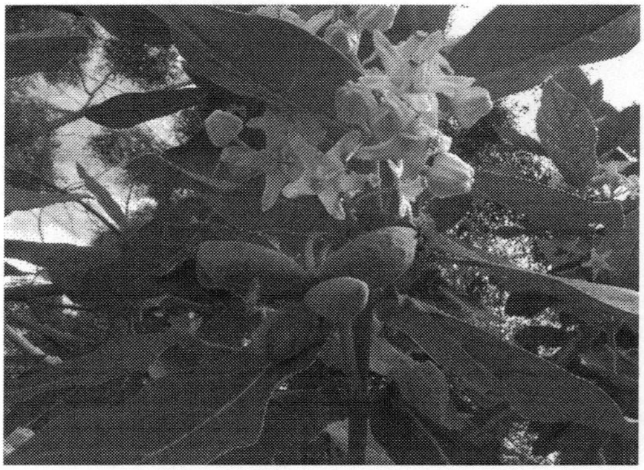

Vernacular Names: *Milk weed, calotropis, swallow-wart, King's crown* (English), *Vellerukku, Vellaierukku* (Tamil), *Tapana, Bhinu* (Sanskrit), *Akanda, Akond* (Bengali), *Erikku* (Malayalam), *Rui* (Marathi), *Ak* (Punjabi), *Arakha* (Odia), *Jilledu* (Telugu), *Ekkegida, Ekka* (Kannada), *Madar, Aak, Akavana* (Hindi), *Aakado* (Gujarati), *Akand, Akan* (Assamese), *Acka* (Kashmiri).

Botanical Description: A small to medium-sized perennial shrub, grows up to 6 m. in height. Stem simple, rarely branched, woody at base. All parts of the plant exude, white milky latex when cut or broken. Bark thick, fibrous, scaly, deeply, fissured, when old, grey to light brown. Leaves simple, opposite-decussate, ovate to obovate with 4-6 pairs of sub-opposite nerves prominent on the abaxial surface. Inflorescence a dense multiflowered, umbellate cyme arising from the nodes, axillary or terminal, flowers hermaphroditic, pentamerous, calyx 5-lobed, shortly. Stamens 5, inserted at the base of the corolla. Fruits consist of green, spongy ovoid up to 16 cm long, 11 cm wide. Seeds many flat obovate, with silky white pappus.

Flowering and Fruiting: September - January

Distribution: Throughout India, Afghanistan, Thailand, Nepal, Pakistan, Ethiopia, Myanmar, Nigeria, Vietnam, Kenya, Kuwait, Iran, Iraq, Africa, Bangladesh, Saudi Arabia, Yemen, Algeria, Sri Lanka, China, Malaysia and Philippines.

Propagation: By seeds, stem cuttings and root cuttings.

Parts Used: Whole plant

Phytochemical Constituents: The whole plant contains trematol, octacosanoic acid, semiarenone, terpenoids, a norditerpenyl ester, calopfriedelenyl, calotropursenyl acetate, calotropternyl ester oleanene triterpenes like calotropoleanyl ester, procerleanol A and B, and cardiac glycosides calotropin, uscharin, calactin, calotoxin and calotropogenin, cardenolides, anthocyanins. The root bark contains α-amyrin, β-amyrin, β-sitosterol, lupeol and flavanols like quercetin-3-rutinoside. The plant yields various types of compounds such as alkaloids, resins, anthocyanins, tannins, sterol, triterpinoids, cardenolide, proteolytic enzymes in latex, flavonoids, cardiac glycosides, saponins. The leaves contain calotropin, calotropagenin, ursosolic acid, cardenolides, amyrin, β-sitosterol, amyrin acetate. The latex contains calactin, uscharin, trypsin, calotropin, caoutchouc, calotoxin, proceroside, syriogenin, uzarigenin and voruscharin. The root bark contains triterpenes, a new norditerpenyl ester, named calotropterpenyl ester, pentacyclic triterpinoids, calotropursenyl acetate, calotropfriedelenyl acetate, mundarol isovalerate, quercetin-3-rutinoside and akundarol isovalerale. The flowers contain sterol, calotropin, calactin, flavonoids, queretin-3-ratinoside, calotoxin, calotropin, polysaccharides with D-arabinose, calotropagenin, glucosamine, glucose and L-rhamnose, 3-proteinase, calotropain (protease), proceroside, proceragenin, lupeol, uscharin, taraxast-20 (30)-en-3-4-methyl-3-pentenoate), syriogenin, gigantin, isogiganteol, giganteol, uzarigenin, uscharidin, 3-thiazoline cardenolide, a-calotropeol, a-lactuceryl acetate, a-lactuceryl isovalerate, 3-epimoretenol and vorusucharin a-calotropeol.

Medicinal Uses: The root bark is used as anthelmintic, laxative, expectorant, depurative and febrifuge. It is used in treating asthma, dyspepsia and bronchitis. The plant is very largely used in treatment of leprosy, elephantiasis and chronic eczema. Leaves are used to cure swellings, paralysis, arthralgia and fevers. Flowers are used in treatment of catarrh, asthma, tumours, anorexia and inflammations. The plant is also used in treatment of jaundice, piles, disorders of spleen, liver and abdomen, and possess antibacterial, antioxidant, anti-inflammatory, antifungal, antipyretic, analgesic activity. It is also used as an abortifacient, treats internal worms, and performs insecticidal, anti-ulcer, anti-fertility and larvicidal activity. Dried root and dried latex is used as an antidote for snake poisoning. They are used in hepatoprotective activity, and perform antidiarrhoeal, antimalarial activity, anticonvulsant, antinociceptive activity. The latex is used to treat dysentery, leprosy, bronchial asthma and skin disorders and can act as carminative, abortifacient, spasmogenic, antisyphilitic, antirheumatic, diaphoretic, mulluscide agent. Roots in the form of paste are applied to cure toothache. The flowers powder mixed with black pepper is ingested to treat snake bite and cholera.

Poisonous Parts: Latex and leaves.

Toxic Constituents: Calotropin and calactin.

Poisonous Symptoms: Accidental contact of milky juice with eyes causes severe inflammation, swelling and redness. Latex and leaves causes diarrhoea and abortion in pregnant livestock. Intake of latex is fatal, and causes damages to eyes leading to blindness. It is also utilized as fish poison.

Cannabis Sativa L.

Family : Cannabaceae

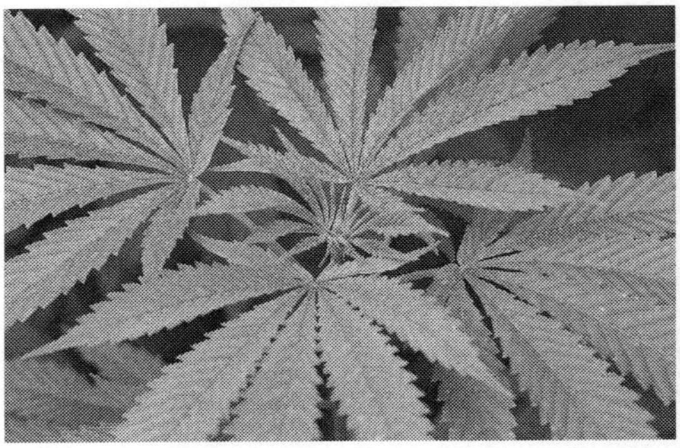

Vernacular Names: *Wild Hemp, Gallowgrass, Hep, Marijuana* (English), *Ganja, Bhang, Charas* (Hindi), *Bahuvadini, Banga, Bhanga* (Sanskrit), *Ganja* (Manipuri), *Bhangi, Bhangigida* (Kannada), *Ginjilachilachi, Cherukanchava* (Malayalam), *Bhang* (Marathi), *Alatam, Ganja, Ganja chedi, Ananta muli* (Tamil), *Bangiaku, Gaanja chettu, Bangiaaku* (Telugu).

Botanical Description: A dioecious, annual and herbaceous 2-5 m high. The leaves are palmately divided into 3-7 narrow, toothed segments. The stems are rough and scabrous and the inner bark is fibrous. The plant is normally a dioecious species, with male and female flowers on separate plants, but sometimes bisexual plants occur, female flowers are in greenish leafy spikes, male flowers are yellowish, tiny, and borne in auxillary clusters, fruit is an achene, hard, one-seeded fruit that remains closed at maturity.

Flowering and Fruiting: Throughout the year

Distribution: USA, India, Mexico, Brazil, Pakistan, China, Bangladesh, Thailand, Africa, The Pacific Islands and Colombia.

Propagation: By seeds

Parts Used: Leaves, whole plant and seeds.

Phytochemical Constituents: The plant contains cannobigerol, cannabigerovarin, cannabichromene, cannabidiolic acid, cannabidiol, cannabidiol-C4, cannabidivarin, cannabidivarinic acid, cannabidiorcol, tetrahydrocannabinolic acid A, tetrahydrocannabinolic acid B, Cannabicyclolic acid, cannabicyclovarin, cannabicyclol, cannabidiol monomethylether, cannabidiol, cannabigerolic acid, cannabigerol, cannabigerolic acid monomethylether, cannabigerol monoethylether, cannabichromenic acid, cannabichromevarinic acid, Delta-9-tetrahydrocannabinolic acid-C4, Delta-9-tetrahydrocannabinol-C4, Delta-9-tetrahydrocannabivarinic acid, Delta-9-tetrahydrocannabivarin, Delta-9-tetrahydrocannabircolic acid, Delta-8-tetrahydrocannabinol acid, cannabielsoin, cannabitriol, cannabitriolvarin, Dehydrocannabifuran, cannabifuran, cannabicitran, cannabichromanon and cannabiripsol. The plant yields myrcene, terpens, sesquiterpenes, limonene, Trans-caryophyllene and caryophyllene-oxide.

Medicinal Uses: The leaves are used to cure malarial fever, dysentery, skin ailments, diarrohea, convulsions, tetanus, otalgia, abdominal disorders, gonorrhoea, insomnia, hydrophobia and colic. Its excessive use causes dropsy, dyspepsia, cough, insanity, impotence, restlessness and melancholy. The bark is used as a tonic to cure hydrocele, haemorrhoids and inflammations. The resin is smoked to cure hiccough and bronchitis. It is useful in treating asthma, whooping cough, insomnia, sick headaches, dysuria, sick headaches, mania, neuralgia, migraine and in relieving pain in dysmenorrhoea and menorrhagia. Medicinally, Indian hemp has been used in the treatment of diseases and health problems such as AIDS/HIV, eye problems glaucoma, cachexia, treatment of pain, convulsion, insomnia, asthma, muscle spasticity, depression and hypertension. The plant is used as a shampoo and for other cosmetic purposes.

Poisonous Parts: Entire parts, but highest toxicity in flower and stalks.

Toxic Constituents: Cannabinon, cannabinol and cannabin, resins cannabidiol, cannabinolic acid, cannabinoids, cannabigerol, cannabicylol and tetrahydrocannabinol isomers.

Poisonous Symptoms: Intake of flower and stalks causes delusions, hallucinations, poor coordination, coma exhilaration and blurred vision.

Carica Papaya L.

Family: Caricaceae

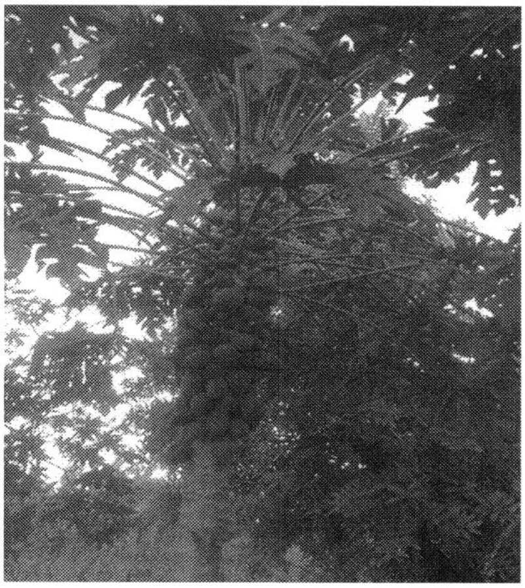

Vernacular Names: *Papaw, Papaya, Papaya tree* (English), *Papeya* (Bengali), *Papita, Papaia* (Hindi), *Papai, Papaya, Popai, Pappayi* (Marathi), *Erand karkati* (Sanskrit), *Pappali* (Tamil), Omakai, Omakaya, Kappalam, Karamooza (Malayalam), *Bappayi pandu* (Telugu), *Amrutbhanda* (Odisha), *Bappayi, Papita* (Punjabi), *Pharangi* (Kannada), *Papaya, Papai* (Gujarati).

Botanical Description: Tree-like plant, 2-13 m in height, usually unbranched, although sometimes branched due to injury, containing white latex in all parts. Stem cylindrical, 12-35 cm in diameter, hollow with prominent leaf scars. Leaves spirally arranged, clustered near apex of trunk, petiole up to 1.2 m long, hollow, greenish or purplish-green, lamina orbicular, 26.77 cm in diameter, palmate, deeply 7-lobed, glabrous, prominently veined, lobes deeply and broadly toothed. Flowers tiny, yellow, funnel-shaped, solitary or clustered in the leaf axis. Male flowers on long hanging panicles with 10 stamens in 2 rows, corolla tube is slender, about 2 cm long. Female flowers 3-5 cm long large functional pistil, no stamens, ovoid-shaped ovary. Fruit is indehiscent, obovoid, 10-40 cm long, fleshy and yellowish or yellow-orange. Seeds numerous, small, black, round, covered with gelatinous aril.

Flowering and Fruiting: Throughout the year.

Distribution: The plant is commonly grown in India, Malaysia, Pakistan, Bangladesh, Mexico, Nigeria, West Indies, Sri Lanka, Philippines, Indonesia, Australia, Central America, Egypt, Kenya, New Zealand, French, Paraguay, Colombia, Cuba, Haiti, Argentina, Peru, Jamaica, Sudan, Thailand, Hawaii, Brazil and throughout the world.

Propagation: Seeds

Parts Used: Leaves, fruits, bark, seeds and latex.

Phytochemical Constituents: The plant contains flavonoids, alkaloids, carbohydrates, triterpenes, cardiac glycosides, anthraquinones and phlobatinins. The leaves contain many active components such as papin, tocopherol, carpinine, carpaine, vitamin C and E, ascorbic acid, flavonoids, chymopapain, cystatin, glucosinolates and cyanogenic-glucosides. It also yields tannins, saponins, flavonoids, alkaloids, glycosides, phenols and steroids. The latex is a rich source of four cysteine endopeptidases namely chymopapin, papain, caricain and glycylendopeptidase. The shoots contain kaemferol and myricetin. The fruits yield Bcarotene, crytoxanthin, Linalool and 4-terpinol. The roots contain carposide. The unripe fruit yield chymopapain and papain. The seeds contain papain, carpine, benzyl isothiocynate, bactericidal aglycone, chymopapain, aglycoside, sinigrin, isothiocyanate, papaya oil, carpasemine and the enzyme myrosin.

Medicinal Uses:

The *C.papaya* possesses anticancer, antiviral, antioxidant, anti-inflammatory and antimicrobial potentialities. It is used to treat several ailments such as asthma, wounds, tumours, nervous pain. The seed is utilized for intestinal worms, infection and various types of wounds. The root is used in bronchitis, cough, respiratory disorders, syphilis and hemorrhoids. The unripe fruit is used as a cure for ulcer, diuretic importance, mild laxative and to stimulate lactation. The leaf extract is used to treat Dengue fever. It is used as antidiabetic, anti-inflammatory, antihypertensive, antihyperlipidemic, antiparasitic, antimicrobial, antiseptic agent. It is used to treat nervous pains and burn wound healing. The seed paste is used to manage stimulation of menstruation, abortion, and can be used as anthemintic, antifungal, stomachic, anti-inflammatory and analgesic agent. Green fruits are used to treat constipation, high blood pressure, dyspepsia, general debility, amenorrhoea, stimulate reproductive organs and expel worms.

Poisonous Parts: Latex and seeds.

Toxic Constituents: Carpine and papain.

Poisonous Symptoms: Externally, the latex is an irritant to the skin, dermatogenic and a vesicant. Internally, it causes dangerous gastritis. Few people are allergic to the pollen, the latex and the fruit and even the enzyme papain has its negative effects. The acid fresh latex can cause severe vesication and conjunctivitis. Plentiful consumption of papaya can cause carotenemia. Intake of seeds or unripe fruits causes abortifacient activity on both humans and livestock.

Cascabela Thevetia (L.) Lippold
Family: Apocynaceae

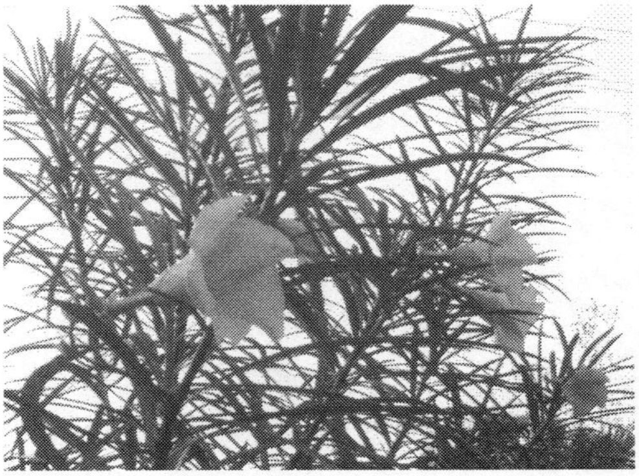

Vernacular Names: *Yellow olender, Exile troe, Exilc oil plant, lucky nut-tree* (English), *Ponnarali, Thiruvachi poo, Majalaleri, Pachaiyalari* (Tamil), *Suicide tree, Pilakaner* (Hindi), *Pachaganneru* (Telugu),

Manja areli, Pachchareli (Malayalam), *Kadukasi, Kanogalu* (Kannada). *Ashvaghna, Haripriyam, Ashvamaraka, Ashvantaka, Shatakunda, Ashvaghna* (Sanskrit), *Chin karabt, Haldi korubi, Koklaphul* (Benhgali).

Botanical Description: Small evergreen plant species of shrub to 4-8m in height with milky juice stems scaled with scars of fallen leaves. Leaves alternate, linear - lanceolate, 11-16 x 0.73 cm. Inflorescence a terminal cyme of 2-3 flowers bisexual, regular, 5 merous, bright yellow. Calyx-lobes 5, unequal, shortly united, corolla yellow, 5.1 cm across, funnel - shaped. Stamens 5, at the throat of narrow tube. Ovary depressed conic, 2.1mm, 2-1- cular, style 1.6mm. Fruit a depressed - globose to turnip-shaped drupe 3-4.2 cm diameter, yellowish green, ripening black, 2-4 seeded within the stony endocarp feeds obovide, brown.

Flowering and Fruiting: Throughout the year.

Distribution: Native of Tropical America, India and Mexico.

Propagation: By seeds and stem cutting.

Parts Used: Leaves, bark, root and seeds.

Phytochemical Constituents: The root and seed contain peruvoside, thevetin A, thevetin B, Cardiotonic glucosides. Peruvonsidic acid, Thevetoxin, Glucosides thevetin, Nerlifolin, ruvoside, alkaloids, flavonoids, steroids, tannins, saponins, anthocyanins, phenolics, fatty acids, coumarins.

Medicinal Uses: Bark and leaf decoction is useful to treat intermittent fever. The plant possess antibacterial and antifungal properties. A leaf decoction is taken to loosen the bowels, as an emetic, and is said to be an effective treatment for antipyretic. The root is used to cure cough, bronchitis and skin diseases. The seed oil is applied externally to treat skin disorders. The seeds act as a contact poison; mashed with a soap solution they are used as an insecticide. It is also used as a febrifuge. The roots are made into a paste which is applied to tumors. The seeds are also utilized to treat dropsy, rheumatism and purgative. The leaves are used as a laxative, narcotic and purgative and can treat vomiting. The crushed seed is useful as insecticide. Bark is a bitter tonic, febrifuge, and is useful in treating various kinds of intermittent fever.

Poisonous Parts: Whole plant, specially latex.

Toxic Constituents: Thevetin A and thevetin B, eight cardiac glycosides as thevetin, thevetoxin and neriifolin.

Poisonous Symptoms: The active principles are cardiac glycosides of the cardenolide type. Seeds are highly poisonous; used for suicide or homicide purpose. Seeds are used to poison and kill enemy's livestock. Intake of seeds cause vomiting, slow irregular pulse, purging drowsiness, dilation of pupils, burning and numbing sensation in mouth and throat.

Cassia Occidentalis L.

Family : Caesalpiniaceae

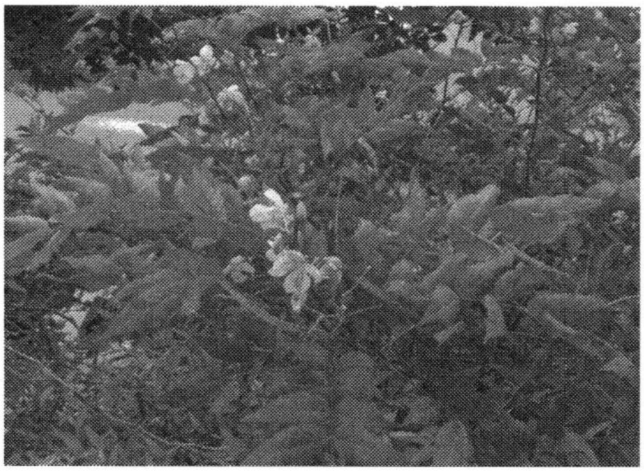

Vernacular Names: *Coffee senna, Stinking weed, Negro coffee* (English), *Kasmard, Kasamardah* (Sanskrit), *Kasondi, Barikasaumdi* (Hindi), *Oolan Takara, Ponnaian, Ponnavaram, Ponnariviram* (Malayalam), *Kattuvuri, Nattam takarai, Ponnavarai, Peravarai* (Tamil), *Kasinda* (Telugu), *Doddaagace* (Kannada).

Botanical Description: An erect, annual herb or under shrub with loosely spreading branches, grows up to 2 m in height, 3-5 pairs. Leaves pinnately, compound, paripinnate with in short pedunculated racemes. Flowers yellow; fruits cylindrical or compressed, transversely septate glabrous 8-15 cm long. Pods containing 10-30 seeds. Seeds ovoid, compressed, smooth, hard and shining dark, pale brown or dark olive green.

Flowering and Fruiting: September-January

Distribution: Throughout India, Sri Lanka, Burma and tropical America.

Cultivation: By seeds

Parts Used : Leaves, roots, flowers and seeds.

Phytochemical Constituents: The whole plant contains emodin, aloe emodin, anthrones, apigenin, achrosin, anthraquinones, cassiollin, campesterol, chryso-obtusin, aurantiobtusin, chrysoeriol, chrysophanol, chrysophanic acid and chrysarobin, free physcion, 1,1-bi-4, 4′,5, 5′-tetrahydroxy-2, 2′-dimethyl anthraquinone, the flavon meterucinol-7-0-α-L-rhamnoside, tetrahydroanthracene derivatives, germichrysone, occidentallins A & B, sennoside, anthraquinone glycosial, fatty oils, flavonoid glycosides, polysaccharides, tannins, galactomannan. The leaf contain glycosides, carbohydrates, anthraquinones, steroids, flavonoids, phytoserols, saponins, cardiac glycosides, guns, mucillages alkaloids, amino acids, proteins, sterols and phenolic compounds, polyphenolics. The seeds contain 1,4,5-trihydroxy-7-methoxy-3-methylan thraquinone, 1,8-dihydroxy-2-methylanthraquinone, physicon, rhein, aloe-emodin, glucose, N-methylmorpholine, chrysophanol, glucosides of compesterol, β-sitosterol and galactomannan.

Medicinal Uses: The plant can perform antidiabetic, antibacterial, antifungal, hepatoprotective, antidiabetic, anticancerous, anti-mutagenic, anti-inflammatory, antimalarial, antiplasmodial, anticarcinogenic activity. The leaves of the paste is externally applied to treat skin disorders, fever, ringworm, cutaneous diseases, itch, wound healing, sores, throat infection and bone fracture. The decoction or powdered leaves serve as an analgesic, antiviral, antiparasitic, carminative, antipasmodic, antiseptic, diaphoretic, febrifuge, laxative, vermifuge, purgative, insecticidal, sudorific, emmenagogue, immunostimulant and anti-hepatotoxic agent. The plant is useful as a tonic, expectorant, diuretic and febrifungal. The plant is also useful for treating typhoid, hematuria, sore eyes, leprosy, disorder of hemoglobin and asthma. It is used as anti-allergic, anti-inflammatory agent, anti-lipidperoxidant, antidote of poisons, blood purifier, and a medication for the treatment of liver disorders. The seeds are used to treat fever, leprosy, cough, ulcers, and can serve as diuretic, bitter, arid, expectorant, febrifuge, and purgative, and they are useful for treating bronchitis, dyspepsia, flatulence, whooping cough and convulsion.

Poisonous Parts: Leaves, seeds, roots and fruits.

Toxic Constituents: Alkaloids, emodin, toxalbumins, glycosides and anthraquinones.

Poisonous Symptoms: Leaves and pod intake by livestock causes gastroenteritis. Accidental intake of seeds and fruits by humans causes vomiting, nausea, diarrhoea, uneasiness and dark brown urine.

Catharanthus Roseus (L.) Don

Family : Apocynaceae

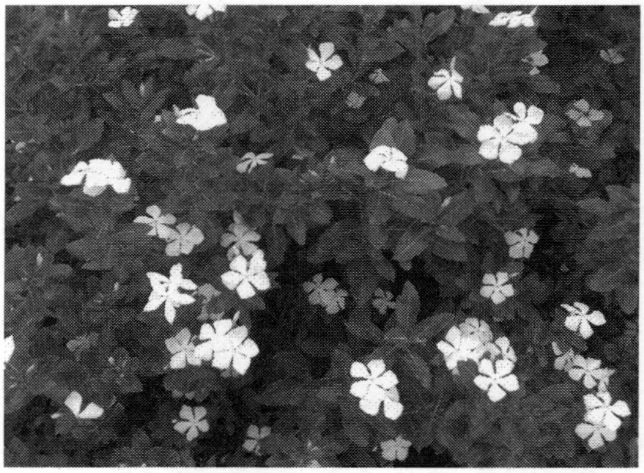

Vernacular Names: *Cape periwinkle, Rose periwinkle, Rosy periwinkle, Old maid, Madagascar periwinkle* (English), *Sada bahar, Baramassi* (Hindi), *Nityakalyani* (Sanskrit), *Billaganeru* (Telugu), *Nityakalyani, Ushamalari* (Malayalam), *Kasikanigale, Nityamallige* (Kannada), *Rattanjot* (Punjabi), *Nithiyakalyani, Sudukattumallikai* (Tamil), *Nayantara* (Bengali).

Botanical Description: An erect herbaceous perennial, grows up to 90 cm, stem erect. Leaves oval to oblong, 2.5-9.0 cm long and 1.1-3.6 cm broad, glossy green, hairless, with a pale midrib and a short petiole 1.1-1.9 cm long. Flowers born on axills in pairs. There are three flower colour types, white, pink and pink-eyed. Calyx with 5 sepal, green, linear, corolla tube is cylindrical with 5 petals rose-purple or white with rose purple spot in the centre. Flowers white to dark pink with a darker red centre, with a basal tube 2.7-3.2 cm long and a corolla 2.2-5.1 cm diameter with five petals like lobes. The fruits are a pair of follicles 2.1-4.2 cm long and 3.1mm broad. Seeds many, minute, blackish brown.

Flowering and Fruiting: Throughout the year

Distribution: Native to Madagascar, West Indies, Sri Lanka, Philippines, Mozambique, South Vietnam, Africa, Southern Europe, India, Jamaica and Australia. It is cultivated in Karnataka, Tamilnadu, Assam, Madhya Pradesh, Gujarat and West Bengal.

Propagation: By seeds

Parts Used: Whole plant

Phytochemical Constituents: The whole plant contains vincoside, catharanthin, reserpine, serpentine, leurosine, monomeric indole alkaloids, α-methylene indines, dihydroindoles, bisindole, 2-acyl indoles, oxindole, vinblastine, vincristine, isovincoside, vindolinine, vincolidine, lochrovicine, asmalicine, loctonerine, vindoline, perivine, perividine, pericalline, periformyline, tetrahydroalstonine, rovidine, leurosidine, leurosivine and carosine. Vincristine, vincaleukoblastine, tabesonine, tryptophan, tryptamine, secologanine, strictosidine.

Medicinal Uses: The plant is used as antidiabetic, diuretic, anthelmintic, antioxidant, tonic, anticancerous, antimicrobial, antihypertensive, antidysenteric, antifibrillic, haemorrhagic and tranquillising agent. It is also known for its antifungal, antiviral, antitumor, anti-diabetic, stomachic, antidiuretic, antifertility, antimalarial, cytotoxic, anti-inflammatory, animal repellent activity, cardiotonic, anti-mutagenic, antiseptic, antihyperglycemic, antispasmodic, antihypetensive, antineoplastic, antioxidant and insecticidal properties. The plant is used to treat childhood leukemia, testicular cancer, cancerous tumors, prevention of cancer, reduce high blood pressure, nose bleeding through external application, mouth ulcers and sore throat. The leaves are used in curing menorrhagia, diabetes and wasp stings. Root is useful as stomachic, sedative, hypotensive, tonic and tranquilliser. Patients with high blood pressure and cancer made to drink the root powder mixed with hot water. They are used to treat muscle pain, depression of central nervous system and wasps stings. It is used in case of nose bleed and bleeding gums. It is also used internally for hypertension, gastritis, loss of memory, cystitis, enteritis, diarrhoea and raised blood sugar levels.

Poisonous Parts: Leaves, seeds and roots.

Toxic Constituents: Alkaloids

Poisonous Symptoms: The leaves and root juice is poisonous and acts as poison to heart. The other parts are also poisonous when consumed in higher doses.

Cleistanthus Collinus (Roxb.) Benth. ex Hook. f
Family: Phyllanthaceae

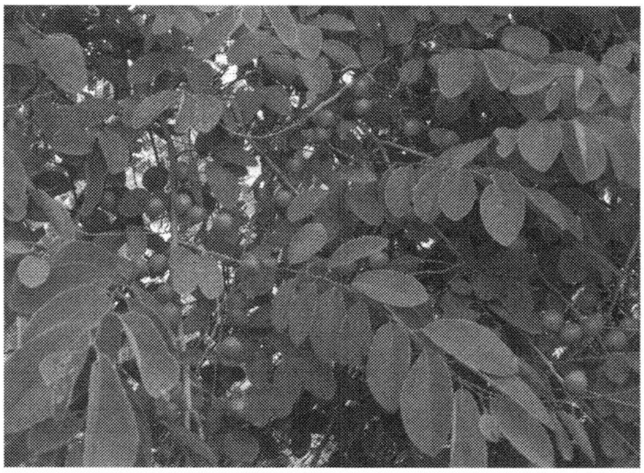

Vernacular Names: *Oduvanthalai, Oduvan, Nillipalai* (Tamil), *Vadisaku, Korshe, Korsi, Kadise* (Telugu), *Kariajuri* (Bengali), *Garari, Garrar* (Hindi), *Garari* (Marathi), *Odugu, Nilappala* (Malayalam), *Korodo* (Odisha), *Indrayava, Kandigam, Kutaja, Nandi* (Sanskrit), *Badedarige, Bodadaraga, Kadagargari* (Kannada).

Botanical Description: Small deciduous free (upto 12m), bark is dark brown, almost black, often with a reddish tinge, rough peeling in rectangular woody scales, leaves are alternate quite entire, leathery, smooth, glabrous, dark green, broadly obovate or elliptic 1.7-4.2 inches long leaf stalk is 6.5 mm long. Flowers are yellowish-green, in small silky hairy clusters in leaf axils. Calyx are ovate -lance shaped. Stamens are 5, filaments united in a column in the centre of the disk, 3 lobed pistillode. Ovary is hairless, styles 3, bifid, capsule is woody, stalkless spherical. Capsules 1.2 x 0.9 cm, glabrous and glossy, brown to dark-brown when ripe.

Flowering and Fruiting: October - February

Distribution: Africa, India, Sri Lanka and Malaysia

Propagation: By seeds

Parts Used: Leaves, stem and bark

Phytochemical Constituents: Lignan lactones, Cleistanthin and Collinusin, Lignins, 3-O-methyl - d-glucose, benzenetriol, 1,6-anhydro - a- D- glucopyranose, heptacosane, 2-hydroxy-7-methoxy - 4, 5-diphenyl - 5 -hindeno, pyrimidine and eicosane, sillane, 1,2,3-Benzenetriol, Thiophene, alkaloids, flavonoids, steroids, terpeniods, tannins, Phlobatannins, glycosides and saponins.

Medicinal Uses: It is a rich source of lignans of which cleistanthin A and B were noted to have the property of anticancer, cytotoxicity and larvicidal activity. Leaf is used for antibacterial and antifungal activities. The leaves are abortifacient and occasionally used for suicidal purposes. The leaf extract is used as anti feedant and insecticide and as washing agent for clearing septic wound. It is also used to cure skin diseases, hoot sores of cattle, and possess antiseptic and piscicidal properties. All parts of the plant are poisonous.

Poisonous Parts: Leaves, bark, roots, outer crust of the capsule.

Toxic Constituents: Cleistanthin A, cleistantihin B, cleistanthin C and cleistanthin D.

Poisonous Symptoms: The bark is poisonous to fish. All parts of the plant are noted to be toxic. Leaves are extremely poisonous; used for suicidal, homicidal purposes. It is also used as cattle and fish poison and for inducing criminal abortion. Leaf extract is used by rural populace and tribals for suicidal purposes and causes nervousness, hypotension and cardiac arythms.

Cryptostegia Grandiflora R.Br.

Family: Asclepiadaceae / Periplocaceae

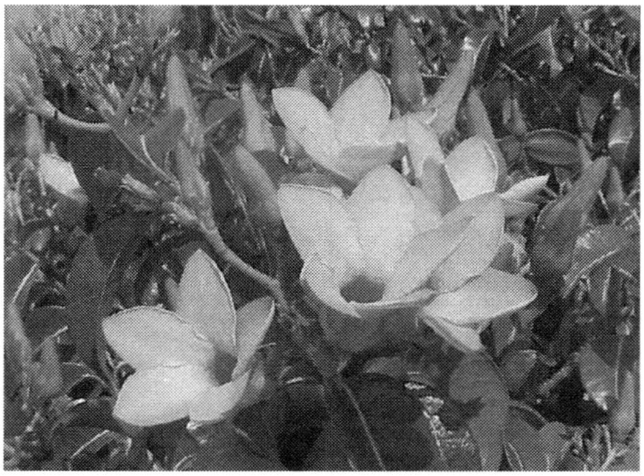

Vernacular Names: *Purple alamanda, Rubber vine* (English), *Rubber kibal* (Hindi), *Hambu rubber gida* (Kannada), *Pala, Palay* (Malayalam), *Vilyati vakundi* (Marathi), *Ganta paala, Rabbarutheega* (Telugu), *Palai, Garudappaalai, Karutappalai* (Tamil).

Botanical Description: A perennial woody climber; grows up to 1-3 m height. The stems are greyish brown with a smooth bark. Milky latex present. Leaves opposite, ovate, smooth, glossy dark green in colour, 6.2–11 cm long, 3.1-5.2 cm wide, thick, oval-shaped with tapered ends, yellow venation. Flowers in pseudumbellate clusters, funnel-shaped, showy, rose-pink. Fruit in spreading, paired follicles. Rigid horn-like seed pods form in pairs, numerous small brown seeds are flat, tight long, white, silky at one end.

Flowering and Fruiting:

Distribution: Madagascar, Australia, Indonesia, USA, Fiji, Egypt, Japan and throughout India.

Propagation: Seeds

Parts Used: Root

Phytochemical Constituents: The plant yielded triterpenoids and phytostenol such as β-sitosterol, β-amyrin, lanosterol, campesterol, stigmasterol, ursolic acid, lupeol, oleic acids, anthocynins, alkaloids, phytoecdysteroids, flavonoids, cardenolides, cryptostigmin I, cryptostigmin II, cryptostimin III, cryptostigmin IV.

Medicinal Uses: The plant decoction is used to cure nervous ailments. The plant also possesses several biological properties such as antitumor, antioxidant, antiviral and antimicrobial. It is also known for its purgative, wound healing, analgesic, anti-inflammatory activity. The paste of the root is applied externally on chest to treat asthma.

Poisonous Parts: Whole plant, particularly thick latex and leaves.

Toxic Constituents: Cardiac glycosides (Cryptostigmin I-IV) and rubber.

Poisonous Symptoms: Some leaves are enough to kill a person or cattle. It causes dry mouth, irritation in the stomach, nausea. The plant is poisonous, and it causes colic, profuse sweating, weakness, muscle twitching and severe cardiac arrhythmias.

Cuscuta Reflexa (Roxb.)

Family: Cuscutaceae

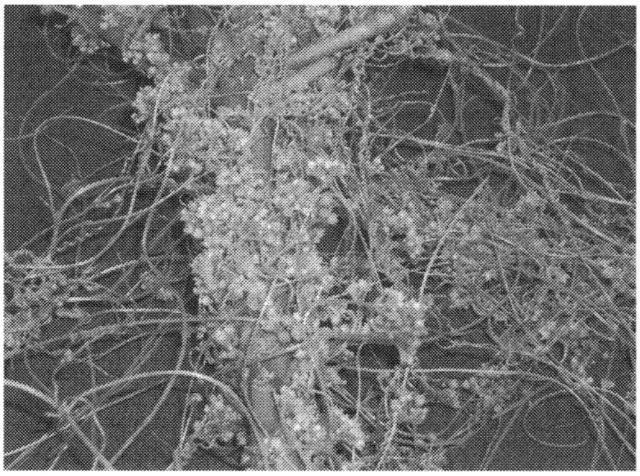

Vernacular Names: *Verillakothan, Sudathari, Kodiyagundal* (Tamil), *Amarlati* (Assamese), *Akashbel, Swarna lata* (Bengali),*Amar Bel, Dodder* (English), *Amar Bel, Amarabela, Akashbel* (Hindi), *Akasavalli, Moodillathali, Akasthamara* (Malayalam), *Uri Sanamacha* (Manipuri), *Nirmali* (Marthi), *Kolanirmuli odisha, Akashbel* (Urdu), *Akasavalli, Amaravalli, Khavalli* (Sanskrit).

Botanical Description: Stem very long, rather stout, closely twining. Stem upto 2.7 mm in diameter, yellowish branched, glabrous. The stems sometimes completely cover the bushes and free crowns. The leaves of the plant have been reduced to minute scales and seeds 3-4, large black and glabrous. Flowers solitary or in umbellate clusters of 205 or in short racemes. Calyx divided almost to the base, lobes 3.1mm. long broadly ovate, globrous and fleshy. Corolla white, stamens 5, filaments very short, overy ovid conical, stigma acute, capsule succulent, 5mm across globose, conical.

Flowering and Fruiting: October - February

Distribution: Bangladesh, Sri Lanka, Malaysia, Bhutan, China and Afghanistan.

Propagation: By seeds and vegetative method

Parts Used: Whole plant and seeds

Phytochemical Constituents: Quercetin, Cuscutine, Cuscutamide, amarbelin, betasterol, cuscutin, Kaempferol, dulcitol, stigmasterol, qurecetin, myricetin, oleanolic acid and coumarin. Myricetin, glucoside, Quercetin-3-0-galactoside, Kaempferol-3-0-galactoside, Quercetin-3-0-galactoside, Isorhamnetol, Azaleatin, Linolenic acid, Cuscutalin, Amarbelin, Bergenine, Beta stitosterol, Oulcitol, Myricetin glucoside, Myricetin, Maragenin, Luteolin, n-Heptacosane, Cusctumine, n-Octacosane, n-Nonacosane, n-Triacontane, Cuscutic acid A, Cuscutic acid B, Cuscutic acid C, Cuscutic acid D, Coffiec acid p-coumari acid, stigmasterol, Avenasterol, Campesterol, Matrine, Saphoronal, Oleanolic acetate, Oleanolic acid, Sesamin Trihydroxy auran, Propenamide, 7-Propenamide, Daucosterol, Kaempterol-3-0-glucoside. Phenolics and flavonoids.

Medicinal Uses: Several parts of this plant were utilized in non-tribal and tribal medicine for the ailments such as melancholoy, fits and insanity. The plant is bitter in taste, acrid, carminative, tonic, expectorant, aphrodisiac, astringent to the bowels, purifies the blood and cleanses the body. It is helpful in treating jaundice, lessens inflammation, headache, pains in the joints and muscles, disorders of vomiting, spleen. The stems are especially beneficial in treating bilious diseases. The plant also possesses hepatotoxic and anti-tubercular activity. The seeds are used as anodyne, depurative and carminative. The stem is useful in treatment of diseases of eye, heart, and can perform antitumor, antioxidant, antispasmodic, homodynamic, antiviral and anticonvulsant activities. It is used to treat lumbago, paralysis, constipation, flatulence, liver complaints, chronic fevers, hiccough, griping, cough, itching, diphtheria, and to expel hookworms. It can perform antifungal, anthelmintic and anti-inflammatory activities.

Poisonous Parts: Whole plant

Toxic Constituents: Phenolics

Poisonous Symptoms: Plant juice causes depression with nausea, abortion and vomiting. Rural populace and tribals mix the plant with fodder to kill enemy's cattle. Intake of plant by animals causes anorexia, vomiting and purgation in animals. Consumption of plant by pregnant livestock results in abortion.

Datura Metel L.

Family : Solanaceae

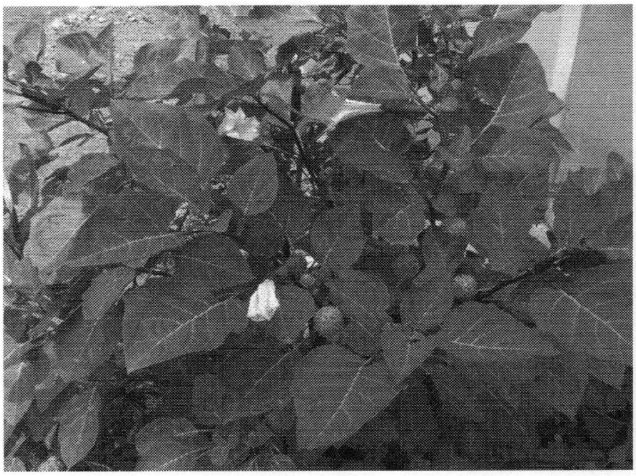

Vernacular Names: *Datura, Downy Thorn-Apple, Devil's Trumpet* (English), *Dhustura* (Sanskrit), *Dhotra-Black* (Marathi), *Dhaturo* (Gujarati), *Kaladhattura, Dhattura* (Hindi), *Ummata, Ummam* (Malayalam), *Karuoomathai, Ummattai* (Tamil), *Dhattura* (Kannada), *Ummetha, Tellavummetta* (Telugu), *Dhatura* (Bengali).

Botanical Description: An annual, ash-green, grows up to 50-90 cm. in height. Leaves simple, uncut. The flowers are strongly scented, with short peduncles, erect and large (15-25 cm.). Flowers large, white, reddish purple or white. The corolla is twice as long as the calyx. Stamens 5;

Fruit globose, pendulous capsule, with small spines. Seeds many, blackish-brown.

Flowering and Fruiting: September - January

Distribution: Throughout India, tropical and sub-tropical Asia, Nigeria, Africa, Tunisia, Algeria, Morocco, Spain, France and Italy.

Propagation: By seeds

Parts Used: Leaves, flowers and root.

Phytochemical Constituents: The whole plant contains carbohydrates, cardiac glycosides, tannins, irredoids, saponins, flavonoids, phenols, glycosides, alkaloids, sugars, triterpenoids, steroids, withanolides, withametelins (1-8), 1, 10-*seco*-withametelin B (9) and 12B-hydroxy-1, 10 *seco*-withametelin B (10), 5′ 7′ dimethyl 6′-hydroxy 3′, phenyl 3α-amine β-yne sitosterol. The leaves contain scopolamine, hyoscyamine, meteloidine and norscopolamine, datumetine, datumeteline, daturibine. The seeds and roots contain alkaloids. The flowers yield hyoscyamine and scopolamine, tigloidine, norhyoscine, apohyoscine, norhyocyamine, tropine, cusiohygrine, DL.scopolamine, normeteloidine, scopine, nortigloidine, tropine, pseudovaleroidine, fastudine, fastunine, tigloylputrescine, fastusinine, 7-hydroxy-3, 6-ditigloyloxytropane (2) datur nolone and fastusic acid.

Medicinal Uses: The plant possesses antioxidant, antimicrobial, antitumor, anti-infectious muscular weakness, analgesic properties, anticholinergic and deliriant properties. The leaf juice is mixed with black pepper and ingested to treat chronic ulcers, asthma and cough.

The plant is also known for its antitumour, anticancerous, ophthalmic, anaesthetic, anthelmintic, antiasthmatic, anticatarrhal and antidiarrhoeal properties. The leaves are sedative, antispasmodic and anodyne properties. They are useful in treating asthma, rheumatism, cough and gastric ulcers.

Poisonous Parts: Entire plant is poisonous. Especially seeds and fruit.

Toxic Constituents: Hyscine, atropine, hyoscyamine and dutarin.

Poisonous Symptoms: Entire plant is narcotic and toxic. Fruits and seeds are poisonous and used for committing offences. Consumption of the leaves, fruits and seeds causes giddiness, staggering, fatal poisoning, dryness of throat, voice becomes unrecognizable and leads to unconsciousness.

Datura Stramonium L.

Family: Solanaceae

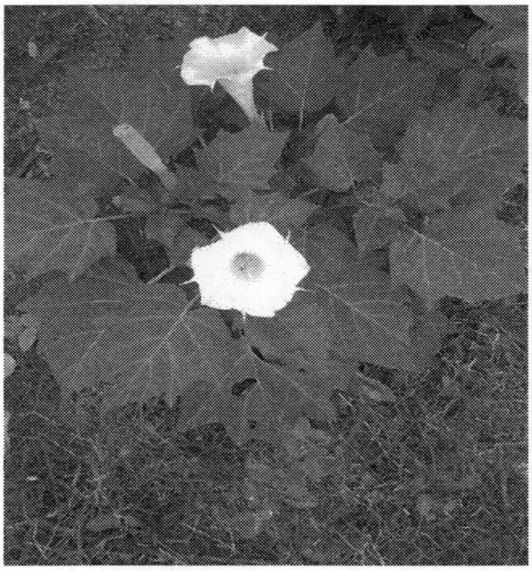

Vernacular Names: *Jimson weed, Mad Apple, Thornapple* (English), *Sadah-Dhatura, Safed-Datura* (Hindi), *Dhatura* (Sanskrit), *Oomatthai, Ummathai* (Tamil), *Maraumman, Ummam* (Malayalam), *Sada dhatura* (Bengali), *Datturamu* (Telugu), *Dhatoria, Dholo dhatura* (Gujrati), *Datura* (Assamese), *Kanaka* (Marathi).

Botanical Description: A large and coarse shrub of about 1-1.5 m in height. The stem is purple or green, smooth, hairless, cylindrical, erect and leafy leaves and single. The alternate leaves are ovate or ovate-cordate in outline. Leaves are cauline and ramal, exstipulate, up to 8.2 cm long and 6.2 cm across. Petiolate, simple, disected, glabrous, acute, unicosted and arranged in reticular venation. The flowers are trumpet-shaped white to creamy or violet and 6.1 to 9.2 cm long with 5 stamens. The flowers are bracteate, pedicellate, ebracteolate, actinomorphic, bisexual, complete, regular pentamerous. The calyx is long, tubular and somewhat are swollen below and very sharply five angled surrounded by 5 sharp teeth. Corolla is funnel shaped. Each flower is replaced by a hard fruit that is dry and spiny, and spheroid-ovoid in shape. Fruits are initially green, but become brown in maturity. They divide into four segments to release the seeds. The seeds are dull, irregular and dark, kidney shaped and flat.

Flowering and Fruiting: Throughout the year.

Distribution: USA, Europe, India, Pakistan, Sri Lanka, Bangladesh, North Africa, South Korea, West Indies, Canada, Hungary, South America, France and throughout the world.

Propagation: By seeds

Parts Used: Leaves, seeds and flowers.

Phytochemical Constituents: The plant contains various types of phytochemicals including alkaloids, tannins, steroids, saponins, glycosides, phenols, flavonoids, carbohydrates and proteins. The larger phytochemicals isolated from *D.stramonium* are tropane, scopolamine, tigloidin, apoatropin, aposcopolamine, atropine, hyoscyamine N-oxide, 64 tropane alkaloids have been detected from *D.stramonium.* 2 new tropane alkaloids, 3-phenylacetoxy-6, 7-epoxynortropane, 7-hydroxyapoatropine, the alkaloids scopoline, 3-tropane, 3-hydroxy-6-tropane, hygrine, pseudotropine, phenylacetoxytropane, hyoscyamine, scopolamine, tropinone, scopine, littorine, 6-hydroxyapoatropine, 3,6-Dihydroxytropane, 3-Acetoxytropane, 3-hydroxy-6-acetoxytropane, Aponorscopolamine, 7-hydroxyhyoscyamine and meteloidine.

Medicinal Uses: *Datura stramonium* has both poisonous and medicinal properties. The plant is used for curing several human maladies including asthma, ulcers, anti-inflammatory, antispasmodic, fever, rheumatism, wounds, inflammation and gout, swellings, bruises, bronchitis, toothache and sciatica. Leaves possess antifungal and antimicrobial properties. Leaf paste is topically applied for skin ailments. The plant can also perform anticancer, antiasthmatic, larvicidal and mosquito repellent activities, and induce pesticide toxicity. It is also used in the treatment of Parkinsonism and hemorrhoids. The leaf paste is externally used for wounds, injuries, pains and bleedings. Juice of flower petal is utilized in ear pain. The seeds are used as a tonic, febrifuge, purgative, tonsil problems, cough, asthma and fever. Seeds are also used for smoking for its narcotic action. The juice of its fruit is applied to the scarp to manage dandruff and falling hair.

Poisonous Parts: All parts of the plant are toxic but the highest amount of the alkaloids is contained in ripe seeds.

Toxic Constituents: It contains a variety of toxic tropane alkaloids such as atropine, hyoscyamine, scopolamine, narcotic cocaine.

Poisonous Symptoms: Headache, speedy and weak pulse, dry, flushed skin, coma, hot, pupil dilation. *Datura stramonium* poisoning is very familiar in India. Common symptoms of *D.stramonium* poisoning include seizures, delirium, mydriasis, agitation, photophobia, paralysis, dry mouth, blurred vision, vomiting, mucous membranes, nausea, decreased bowel, altered mental status, hyperpyrexia, sinus tachycardia, myoclonic jerking, urinary retention, sounds, extreme thirst, hypertension, loss of consciousness, coma, difficulty swallowing and speaking, hyperthermia, decreases in the weight of the liver, significant increases in the levels of red blood cells, white blood cells, hemoglobin, hematocrit, spleen and brain. Tataxia, confusion, psychosis, hallucinations, impaired short-term memory, disorientation, respiratory failure, cardiovascular collapse, dryness of the skin, rapid heartbeat, restlessness and hallucinations. It is a hallucinogenic plant that causes severe poisoning. Consumption of any part of the plant may result in a dangerous anticholinergic reaction that may lead to toxicity and occasionally causes diagnostic problems.

Dioscorea Bulbifera L.

Family: Dioscoreaceae

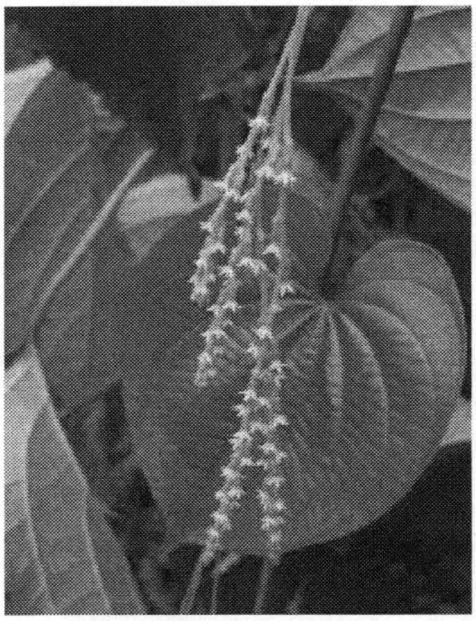

Vernacular Names: *Air potato, Aerial yam, Air yam, Potato yam, Wild yam* (English), *Varahi* (Sanskrit), *Kadu-karanda, Dukkarakand* (Marathi), *Kaachil, Kattukachil, Alanthal, Pannikizhangu* (Malayalam), *Zimikand* (Hindi), *Kukuralu, Ban Alu* (Bengali), *Pannu Pilangu, Pannukkizhangu, Kattu-c-ciraka-valli, Kaattu-k-kaay-valli* (Tamil), *Adavi Dumpa* (Telugu), *Pita Alu* (Odisha), *Ambali Genasu, Negilugonne, Kuntagenasu, Hamdigenasu* (Kannada).

Botanical Description: A twinning perennial herb with minute or absent underground tubers. The climbing stems are rounded, slightly angled, green or purplish-tinged. Stems to 15 m or more in length, terete. The leaves are alternate, attractive, broadly heart-shaped, up to 22 cm long and attached by long petioles. Bulbils many frequent in leaf axils and in inflorescence. Male flower in slender, axillary panicled spikes, pendulous to 17 cm long, bracteoles ovate, acute, perianth light green, tubes 6, stamens 6, female spikes 1-3 together, staminodes 3, ovary triquetrous, 3-locular, ovules 2-per locules, styles 3. Capsule 1.9-2.3 cm long, partially winged.

Flowering and Fruiting: August - October

Distribution: Africa, India, China, Philippines, Malaysia, Japan, Indonesia, Australia, USA, West Indies, Bangladesh, Nigeria, Zimbabwe, Madagascar and Thailand.

Propagation: By tubers

Parts Used: Tubers

Phytochemical Constituents: The plant contains flavonoids, isoflavonoids, terpenoid, saponin, steroid, cardiac glycoside, glycosides, alkaloid, resin, sterol, daucosterol, diosbulbin-B, β-sitosterol, succinic acid, palmatic acid, shikimic acid, 3,5-dimethoxykaempferol, caryatin, catechin, myricetin, myricetin-3-0-β-D-galactopyranoside, hyperoside, Kaempferol, Kaempferol-3-0-β-D-galactopyranoside, vanillic acid, isovanillic acid, epicatechin, neoxanthine, protocatechnic acid, mono-arachidin, stigmasterol, tetracosanoic cid, tristin, violaxanthin, zeaxanthin, behenic acid, caryatin, adenosine, auroxanthin, bafoudiosbulbins A1 and B2. Cyrptoxanthin, demethyl batatasin IV, enolglycoside lucein.

Medicinal Uses: Tubers are used to cure leucoderma, wounds, asthma, anthelonintic, aphrodisiac and expectorant. The tubers are also used as a remedy for dysentery, diuretic, syphilis, piles, ulcers, pain, inflammation, diarrhea. It can exhibit anticancer, antioxidant, antitumour, anti-inflammatory, antidiabetic, antimicrobial, antibacterial activities. The plant is used to treat scrofula, hemorrhoids, diabetic disorders, worm infestations, flatulence, sore throat, gastric cancer and leprosy. The powdered bulbil soaked in water is serviceable in reducing high blood pressure.

Poisonous Parts: Tuber

Toxic Constituents: Disobulbin-D, furano norclerodane diterpenoid, alkaloids, saponins, tannins and diterpenelactone.

Poisonous Symptoms: Tubers consumption in extensive quantities causes paralysis of respiratory system and even death. Eating the aerial tuber causes burning, sting and swelling of the mouth and tongue. Medical attention is needed.

Euphorbia Antiquorum L.

Family: Euphorbiaceae

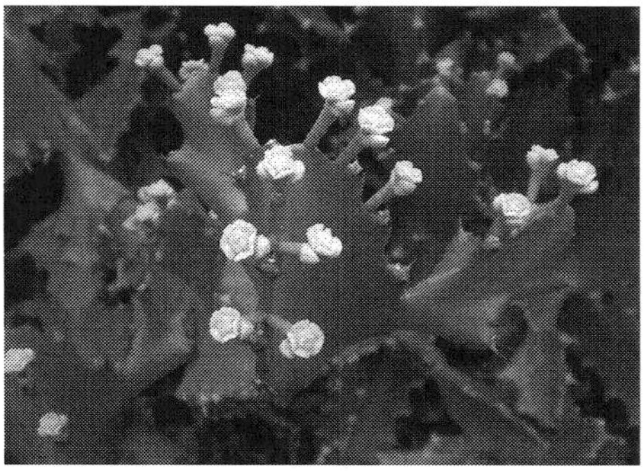

Vernacular Names: *Cactus, Square spurge, Square milk hedge* (English), *Tidhara-sehud* (Hindi), *Caturakkalli, Chatirakkal* (Malayalam), *Thuvar, Tidhari nivadunga, Tidharithor* (Marathi), *Snuhu, Vajrakantaka* (Sanskrit), *Sathurakkalli, Kalli, Kodiravan, Kantiravan, Tiruvargalli* (Tamil), *Mundukalli, Jadekalli, Darekalli, Bontekalli* (Kannada), *Bonthakalli, Peddajemudu, Bonthajemudu, Bommajemudu* (Telugu), *Nerasij, Bojbaran, Sibgach, Tiktasij* (Bengali).

Botanical Description: A wide shrub or small tree, spinous tree, 5-10 m in height, with white latex, branches several curving upwards, stem 5.3-7.5 cm thick green, glabrous, spines paired, sharp 2.6 mm long. Leaves few, borne on the ridges succulent, alternate, apically clustered, petiole very little, leaf blade obovate, margin entire flowers cyathia yellowish-green to pinkish, axillary, cyathia peduncle 2.2-3.1 mm, all cyathia bisexual, anthers pinkish, male flower with only one stamen, filament short, female flower situated alone at the centre of the cyathium, styles 3. Fruit capsules, smooth, obscurely lobed, seeds brown-yellow, globose, smooth.

Flowering and Fruiting: Throughout the year

Distribution: China, India and Sri Lanka.

Propagation: By seed or vegetative.

Parts Used: Root and latex.

Phytochemical Constituents: The plant contains antiquorine A, antiquorine B, taraxerol, terpenoids, triterpenoids, diterpenoids, antiquol A, antiquol B, eupol, taraxerone, beta-amrine, cycloartena, alpha-euphorbol. Latex contains euphol, cycloartenol, β-amyrin, euphorbol, lupenone, euphadienol, triedelin, diacetate, triedelanol, triedelanacetate, lupeol cinnamate, mortenone and ψ-taraxastane-β-antiquorin.

Medicinal Uses: The plant is used to treat toothache, gout, inflammatory disorders, venereal sores, scabies, cough, branchitis, asthma and tuberculosis. It possesses antibacterial, antifungal, antiviral, anti-inflammatory, anthelmintic, antimolluscal, cytotoxic properties. The dried latex is given orally in fewer doses to help clear motion. The root is used to treat constipation, ulcers, colic, otalgia and wounds. The root juice is useful for cough, cutaneous ailments, dropsy and rheumatism. Stem juice is used to treat earache. The latex is used in toothache, purgative, dropsy, nervine disorders, whitlow and cutaneous affection.

Poisonous Parts: Latex

Toxic Constituents: Euphol, euphorbol and euphadienol.

Poisonous Symptoms: 25 ml of latex is given orally causes female infant death. The latex causes vomiting and diarrhoea.

Euphorbia Cyathophora L.

Family: Euphorbiaceae

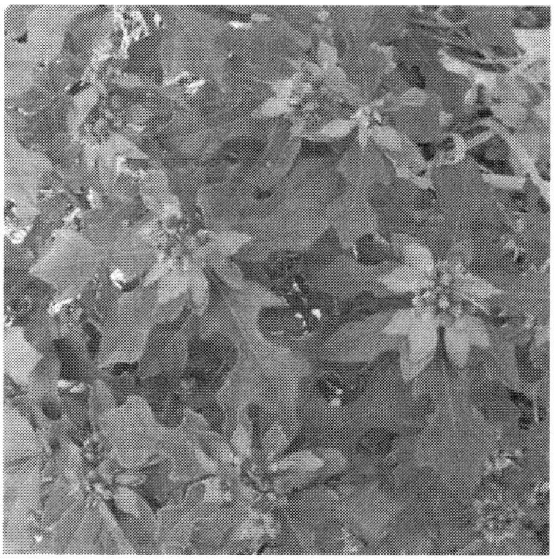

Vernacular Names: *Wild poinsettia, Fire plant, Desert poinsettia, Pointed euphorbia, Mexican fire plant, Pointed-leaf spurge* (English), *Titti phool* (Hindi).

Botanical Description: An erect herb, growing up to 32-80 cm in height. The leaves at the upper end of the stalk close to the cyathium have a striking, scarlet red colour. Alternately arranged leaves are very variable. Leaf stalk is slender 1.2-4.3 cm long. The stalk exudes a toxic milky white sap. The cyathia or fake flowers are placed in clusters at the head of the stalk and are yellowish green. They have no petals, the red colour being part of the immature leaves colouration. The fruits are small, segmented capsules. The mature flower produces 3 oval black seeds. Flowers are yellowish with 1-2 small glands or nectaries and occur in compact in cymes.

Flowering and Fruiting: June - November

Distribution: India, Australia, Pakistan, Bangladesh, Mexico, Thailand, USA, Guatemala, Pana ma, Chile, Bolivia, Argentina and Ecuador.

Propagation: Seeds

Parts Used: Leaves

Phytochemical Constituents: The plant contains various chemical constituents such as flavonoids, alkaloids, tannins, steroids, terpenoids, glycosides, saponins. The leaves contain quercetin and roots yield diterpenoids.

Medicinal Uses: The leaf possesses antimicrobial activity, wound healing activity, hepatoprotective, laxative property, cure skin ailments and antigonorrheae.

Poisonous Parts: Whole plant and latex.

Toxic Constituents: The aerial latex contains glucosides, phorbol esters and alkaloids.

Poisonous Symptoms: A short twig can cause death in children. Dangerous irritation in stomach, mouth and throat. The latex causes diarrhoea and vomiting. In dangerous cases, delirium and dehydration may lead to death. Consumption of the latex and leaves have caused the death of a young children. The milky latex, sticky sap causes severe skin irritation and is toxic to livestock and humans.

Euphorbia Hirta L.

Family: Euphorbiaceae

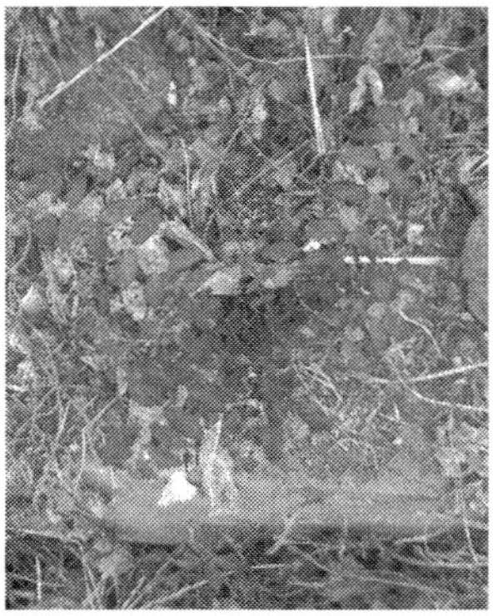

Vernacular Names: *Australian asthma herb, Asthma herb, Snake weed* (English), *Baria Dudhi, Dudhi, Mothi Dudhi* (Hindi), *Barokherni, Barokarni* (Bengli), *Amman pacharisi, Amman - paccarici* (Tamil), *Nanapala* (Telugu), *Nagari, Dughika, Ksira, Nagarjun* (Sanskrit), *Dudhi* (Marathi), *Dhedhi - dudheli* (Rajasthani), *Pakhamba maton* Manipuri), *Nilappala, Nilappaala, Kuzhinagappala* (Malayalam), *Akkigida, Achchedida, Kempuneney* (Kannada).

Botanical Description: A small annual herb spreading upto 75 cm tall, branches ascending, leaves opposite, broadly oblong to elliptic - base obliquely truncate, apex acute, hispid on both side, basically 3-nerved. Cyathia aggregated in single or paired axillary clusters. Inflorescence of several male florets surrounding a solitary female floret enclosed within involucres. Involucre campanulate, 0.8-0.7mm; anther 0.2 mm, ovary 0.9 mm across. Seeds minute, red 4-angled, minutely furrowed. Cyathia aggregated in single or paired axillary clusters.

Flowering and Fruiting: Throughout the year

Distribution: Native to India and Australia, China, Philippines, Africa and Malaysia.

Propagation: By seeds

Parts Used: Whole plant

Phytochemical Constituents: The leaves contain alkanes, terpenoids, phenolic acids, flavonoids, choline sand shikimic, alkaloids, tannins, steroids, glycosides, carbohydrates, saponins, lipid pholabatannins, Resins, sterols, anthraquinone, phenols and acidic compounds.

Medicinal Uses: The leaves are used to cure dysentery, asthma, cough, colic troubles, worms and vomiting. Paste of leaf is applied externally (thrice daily) on the place of scorpion bite. The fresh milky latex is applied on piles, swellings, boils, wounds, epilepsy, miscarriage, warts and in sprains and inflammation. The plant has been noted for anti-inflammatory, antibacterial, antiamoebic, antispasmodic, antioxidant, antidiabetic and antidiarrhoea activities. The plant decoction is used to treat several disorders including diarrhoea, peptic ulcers, intestinal parasites, vomiting, amoebic dysentery, asthma, hay fever, cold, cough, kidney stones, bronchitis, sterility, veneral diseases and menstrual problems. Traditionally, it is used in the remedy of respiratory diseases, bronchial, gastrointestinal disorders, diabetes and in conjunctivitis. It also exhibits analgesic, antipyretic, anti-inflammatory anxiolytic potentialities. The plant is also used as antifungal, sedative, diuretic, anathematic, larvicidal, antidiarrheae agent, and increases electrolytes.

Poisonous Parts: Whole plant

Toxic Constituents: Glycosides, alkaloids, steroids and tannins.

Poisonous Symptoms: The latex causes injuries to eyes. The plant extract has sedative causes on the mucous membrane of the respiratory and genitourinary tract. Consumption of whole plant by animals in large quantity causes vomiting, salivation and nausea.

Euphorbia Milii L.

Family: Euphorbiaceae

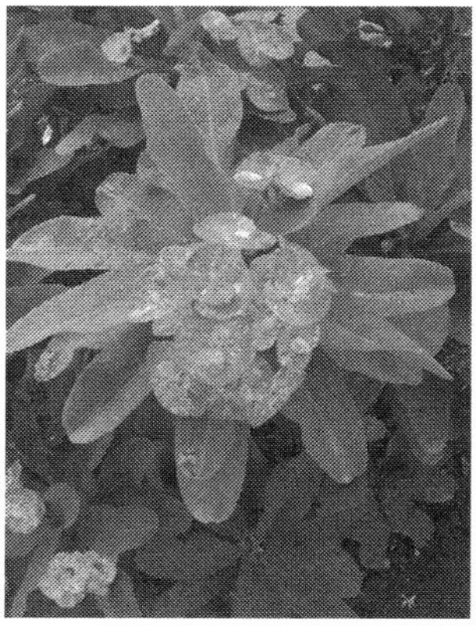

Vernacular Names: *Crown of thorns, Christ thorn, Christ plant, Chirst's plant, Madagascar spurge, Christ cactus, Red crown of thorns* (English), *Kreedakalli, Alakonakalli* (Tamil).

Botanical Description: A bushy, very spiny, succulent climbing shrub, growing to 1.5 m in height, with densely spiny stems are 5-7 sided, greyish-brown, branched and with several prominent grey spines, the erect, slender spines up to 2.8 cm long. The leaves are found chiefly on new growth, and are obovate, up to 3.2 cm long and 1.6 cm broad. The inflorescence is composed of a specialized structure termed a cyathium comprising a cup like involucre, within which is set a solitary much reduced female flower surrounded by 3 male flowers reduced to one stamen. The cyathia are borne in cymes and each cyathium is subtended by 2 colourful bracts.

Flowering and Fruiting: Throughout the year

Distribution: India, Madagascar, Thailand, Pakistan, Nepal, China and Bangladesh.

Propagation: By tip cuttings, v-grafting and seeds.

Parts Used: Latex

Phytochemical Constituents: The plant contains flavonoids, terpenoids, tannins, lupeol, euphol, β-amyrin, β-sitosterol and cycloartenol, dithioteritol, phenyl-methanesultonyl fluroide, trichloracetic acid II, trifluoroacetic acid, β-mercaptoethanol, sulphonic acid II.

Medicinal Uses: The plant exhibits antimicrobial activity, cytotoxic activity, molluscicidal activity. It performs a role in folk medication. It is used to treat warts and cancer. The latex is used to cure hepatitis, sprains and abdominal edema.

Poisonous Parts: Sap

Toxic Constituents: Diterpene esters in milky latex.

Poisonous Symptoms: Milky juice of all parts of the plant is highly poisonous causing swelling, redness, vomiting, nausea, diarrhoea and blisters following contact with skin. The sap causes severe irritation or temporary blindness in eyes and swelling, redness and blisters on skin. Ingestion of the Crown of thorns results in vomiting, abdominal pains, throat irritation and blistering. The plant produces abundant quantities of poisonous milky sap that causes skin irritation.

Euphorbia Neriifolia L.

Family: Euphorbiaceae

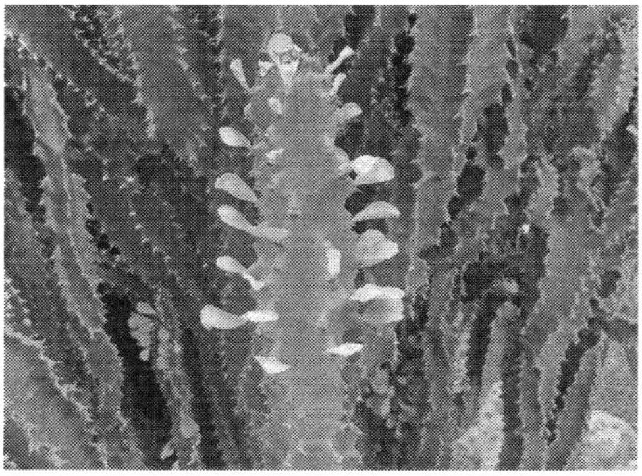

Vernacular Names: *Common Milk Hedge, Indian Spurge Tree, Oleander Spurge, Hedge Euphorbia* (English), *Vijri, Vajra, Snoohi, Svarajana, Patrajnuk* (Sanskrit), *Neya-dungra* (Marathi), *Yelekalli* (Kannada), *Thohar, Sij, Sehund, Patton-Ki-Send* (Hindi), *Ilaikkalli* (Tamil), *Patasiji, Hij-daont, Mansasij* (Bengali), *Akujumudu* (Telugu).

Botanical Description: A large succulent shrub, erect, branched, fleshy, cactus like plant, 3 to 8 m in height, with stipular thorns, leaves succulent, deciduous, 15-30 cm, long, terminal on the branches, waved narrowed into a very short petiole. The order of flowers in a bunch on the plant is cyathium category, means 1 female and many male flowers are found on a same bunch. Female flowers consist of a trichambered ovary. Fruits are 3 chambered and tricoccous.

Flowering and Fruiting: March - May

Distribution: India, Malaysia, Thailand, Philippines, China, Vietnam and New Guinea.

Propagation: By stem cuttings and seed.

Parts Used: Whole plant including latex.

Phytochemical Constituents: The plant yielded nerifoliol, beta-amyrion, taraxerol, euphol, monohydroxy triterpene, neriifolione, cycloarfenol, glut-5-(10)-en-1-one flavonoids, triterpenes, steroidal saponins, tannins, alkaloids, triterpenoidal saponin, sugar, cardenoloids, phenol, terpenoids, saponin, phlobatannins, cardiac glycosides, lignins.

Medicinal Uses: The plant is used to treat fever, abdominal troubles, tumors, piles, leucoderma, enlargement of spleen, anemia, inflammation, chronic respiratory troubles and ulcers. The plant is used as a laxative, carminative and improves appetite. The leaves are used as aphrodisiac, antimicrobial, diuretic, and also utilized in the cure of bronchitis, cold, cough, bleeding piles and in ano-rectal fistula. It is also used in the curing of anal problems like fistula-in-ao and haemorrhoids. The plant possesses hepatoprotective, anti-inflammatory, analgesic, antioxidant, immunomodulatory would healing, antidiarrhoeal, anti-ulcer and antifungal, antibacterial, antiviral, antiarthritic, antiparasitic, antidiabetic, anti-cancer, anticonvulsant, spasmodic and radioprotective properties. Latex is used to treat earache, defrost skin warts and in arthritis. The roots are antispasmodic, and the root mixed with black pepper is applied externally to treat snakebites.

Poisonous Parts: Latex

Toxic Constituents: Triterpenes, nerifolione and cycloartenol.

Poisonous Symptoms: The latex injures eyes and causes dermatitis. The plant is poisonous and skin contact of the sap can cause blistering. The roots and leaves have been utilized as a fish poison.

Euphorbia Nivulia Buch-Ham.

Family: Euphorbiaceae

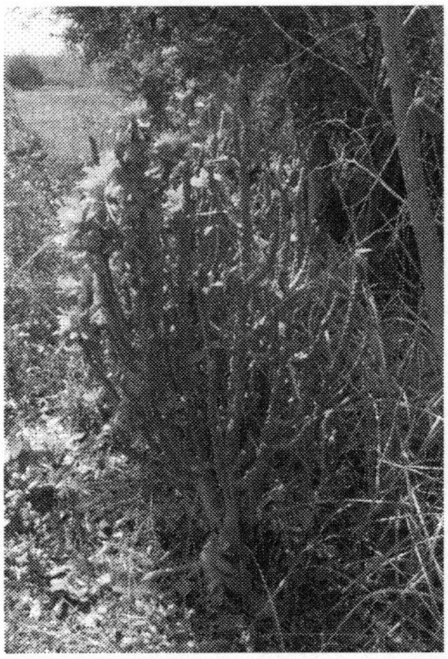

Vernacular Names: *Indian spruge tree, Common milk hedge, Holy milk hedge, Leafy milk hedge* (English), *Katatho-har, Sij, Thor, Senhur* (Hindi), *Adhoguda, Guda, Gandira, Mahavrksha* (Sanskrit), *Ela-calli, Ilakalli, Kallippala* (Malayalam), *Svarasana* (Odisha), *Sij* (Bengali), *Elegalli, Gutagalli, Dundukalli, Dubbakalli* (Kannada), *Akujemu-du, Bonthajamudu, Akukalli* (Telugu), *Nanan-galli, Ilakalli, Manjeri* (Tamil).

Botanical Description: A succulent branched spiny, deciduous tree up to 6-11 m. in height. bark thick, rough. Leaves alternate, sessile or subsessile. Leaf blades obovate-spathulate to oblanceolate, lateral nerves 6-8 pairs. Cyathia in axillary pe-dunculate, cymes of 3 each, towards the tips of the branches reddish, Glands transversely oblong, yellowish. Fruits triradiate, the lobes laterally compressed. Styles stout, united to above the middle. Seeds ovoid-quadrangular, smooth.

Flowering and Fruiting: February-June.

Distribution: India, Pakistan and Burma.

Propagation: By stem cuttings.

Parts Used: Root, bark, stem, juice of leaves and latex.

Phytochemical Constituents: The leaves contain flavonoids, alkaloids, glycosides, proteins, carbohydrates, saponins, terpenes and phytosterols. The plant contains steroids, anthocyanins, terpene and cycloartenol. The bark contains hexacozonate, n-hexacosanol, cycloartenol, euphorbol and euphol. The latex yielded triterpenoid, cycloartenol, cycloeucalenol and cyclonivulial. The stem contains triterpenes.

Medicinal Uses: The leaf juice is useful as diuretic, purgative and is utilized to cure acute asthma. The root, stem, leaf and latex are used to treat diabetes, leprosy, anemia, abdominal ailments, rheumatoid arthritis and oedema. It serves as wound healing, antimicrobial, larvicidal, insecticidal, cytotoxic, haemostatic and hematicidal agent. Latex possesses wound healing, cytotoxic, anti-inflammatory, haemostatic and antiproliferative properties.

Poisonous Parts: Latex or sap.

Toxic Constituents: Triterpenoid, cycloartenol and cyclonivulial.

Poisonous Symptoms: The milky latex or sap is highly toxic and causes intense inflammation of the skin and the eye.

Euphorbia Pulcherrima Willd.

Family: Euphorbiaceae

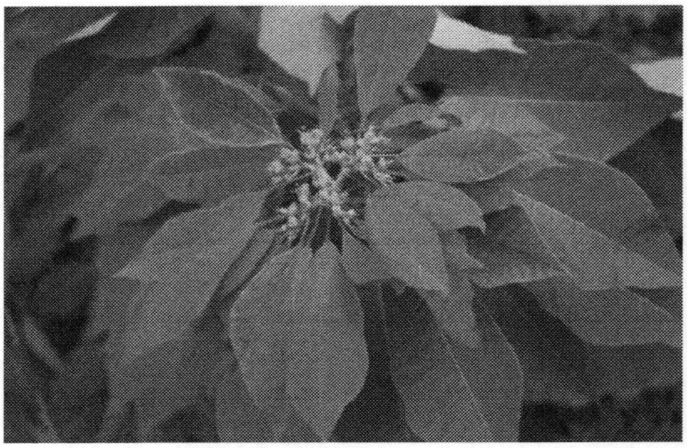

Vernacular Names: *Christ flower, Christmas star, Poinsettia, Christmas flower, Mexican flame leaf* (English), *Pookalli, Ilaipaddi, Mayilkalli* (Tamil), *Lal pate* (Hindi).

Botanical Description: A shrub or small trees, typically reaching a height of 0.5 to 4 m. Dark green dentate leaves 7 to 16.5 cm in length. The coloured bracts, which are greatest often flaming red but can be pale green, orange, pink, white, cream or marbled are often mistaken for flower petals because of their groupings and colours, but are actually leaves. Inflorescence is terminal, involucers are ovoid, about 1 cm long, the margins toothed, each with 1 or 2 large yellow glands.

Flowering and Fruiting: April - November

Distribution: USA, Africa, Australia, England, India, Bangladesh, Pakistan, China, Iran, Spain, Mexico, Chile, Peru, Guatemala, Nepal, Germany, Thailand, Russia, Japan, Egypt, Malaysia and France.

Propagation: By seeds and stem cuttings.

Parts Used: Leaves and flowers.

Phytochemical Constituents: The presence of several classes of phytoconstituents such as steroids, terpenoids, alkaloids, saponins, amino acid, reducing sugar and glycosides. The leaves contain saponins, alkaloids, amilodetrin and formic acid.

Medicinal Uses: The plant cures typhoid, gastro-enteritis, fever and asthma. It is also used to manage emetic, tuberculosis, skin infections, galactagogue and cutaneous problems.

Poisonous Parts: Plant juice

Toxic Constituents: Diterpene esters

Poisonous Symptoms: Latex is irritant to tender skin and mucous surface producing blistering, vomiting, intense gastroenteritis and purgation of bowels accompanied by delirium. Ingestion can lead to mild irritation of the stomach and mouth. Latex is poisonous to livestock. Latex is poisonous and causes irritation in wounds, an allergic reaction in sensitive individuals. It is also mildly irritating to the stomach or skin and may sometimes cause vomiting and diarrhea if eaten.

Euphorbia Tirucalli L.

Family: Euphorbiaceae

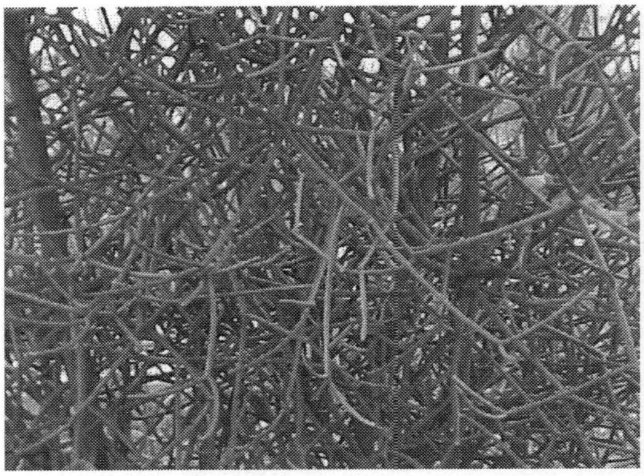

Vernacular Names: *Pencil tree, Indian tree spurge, Milk bush* (English), *Trikantaka, Shatala* (Sanskrit), *Kalli, Tirukalli* (Tamil), *Shera* (Malayalam), *Sehund, Konpol* (Hindi), *Chemudu* (Telugu), *Bantakalli* (Kannada), *Shera* (Marathi), *Lankasij, Latadoona, Ganderi* (Bengali), *Thor-dandalio* (Gujarati).

Botanical Description: A much branched small tree with cylindric or a large shrub up to 5.6 cm tall with erect branches, bark rough, greenish brown, cracked, white latex extraordinarily abundant, sticky and acrid, small linear-oblong leaves, exuding a milky sap when cut branch lets slender, cylindrical, polished, smooth, whorled and modified into phylloclade. Flowers shortly pedicelled, mostly female campanulate, bracteoles many, cocci dark brown, seeds ovoid, smooth.

Flowering and Fruiting: June - October

Distribution: Tropical Africa, India, Brazil, Madagascar, Malaysia and Indonesia.

Propagation: By stem cuttings

Parts Used: Latex, stem and root

Phytochemical Constituents: The plant yielded cardiacglycoside, phenols, anthraquinone, tannins, steroids, alkaloids, flavonoids and diterpenes. The plant also contains terpenes, cycloeupornol, alfa eufor-bol, taraxasterol, *E.tirucallol,* n-hexacosanol, trigliance and terpenic alcohol, β-sitoster-ol, amyrin, euphol, palmitic acid, taraxerol, isoeuphorbol, euphorbinol, trimethyl ellagic acid, tirucallol, tinyatoxin, cycloeuphorde-nol, 4-deoxyphorbol and its ester. The latex contains diterpene esters of the phorbol, 12-deoxyporbol, ingenol ketone euphorone, tirucallol, isoeuphorol, taraxasterol and res-in. The stem contains beta-sitostexotechouc, ellagic acids, campesterol, kaempferol, stig-masterol, methyl ellagic acid, gallic acids, euphol, hentriacontene, hentriacontanol, casuarin, corilagin, euphorbins, euphorene, glucosides, euporcinol and anti-tumor ste-roid 4-deoxy-dhorbol ester. Root contains taraxerone, euphorbol, cycloartenol, tinya-toxin and hexacosanonate. Bark contains triacetate, taraxerone, euphorbol, hexacosan-ate, euphorginol = taraxer 14-en-6-01 and ingenol.

Medicinal Uses: The stem of the decoction is used to treat asthma, leprosy, dropsy, purgative, whoop-ing cough, gonorrhea, carminative, jaundice, tumours, colic and stone in the bladder. Juice of the plant is utilized in the cure of jaundice, asthma, whooping cough and enlargement of spleen. The root is used for colic pains and vesicant. The stem latex is used in the treatment of toothache, rheumatism, warts, skin ailments, asthma, earache, cough, intestinal worms, syphilis, laxative, sarcoma, skin tumours, epithelioma and verrucae. The plant is also known for its antimicrobial, hepatoprotective, antifungal, anti-arthritic, anti-mutagenic, antimalarial, antioxidant, larvicidal, molluscicide, insecticidal, antiparasitic and antiarthritic properties. Stem, bark and leaves possess insecticidal and antibacterial properties. Latex is used to manage anticancer activity, larvicidal activity, proteolytic activity and molluscidal potentialities. The stem is used to cure blood complaints, whooping cough, asthma, dyspepsia, leprosy, syphilis, neuralgia and stomachic.

Poisonous Parts: Milky sap (Latex)

Toxic Constituents: Essential oil, amino acids, alkaloids, cyanogenic glycerides, plant acids, proteins, peptides, saponins, terpenes, tranocoumarins and poly-acetylene compounds.

Poisonous Symptoms: The milky sap is toxic and causes severe skin irritation, redness, mucosa and a burning sensation, contact with the eyes may cause difficult pain and in some cases temporary blindness for many days. Death of a man through hemorrhagic gastroenteritis occurs due to ingestion.

Excoecarica Agallocha L.

Family: Euphorbiaceae

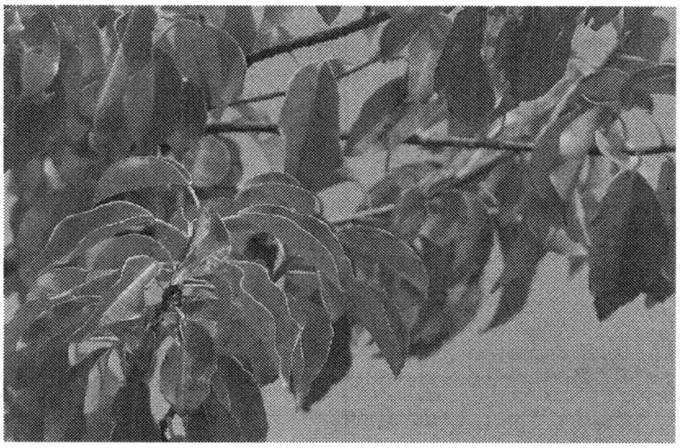

Vernacular Names: *River poison tree, Blinding tree, Milky mangrove, Blind-your-eye* (English), *Gangiva, Tejbala* (Hindi), *Koomatti* (Malayalam), *Geoa, Gneoa* (Bengali), *Tilla, Tella, Chilla* (Telugu), *Hara, Haro, Hanrogida* (Kannada), *Geva* (Marathi), *Guan* (Odisha), *Agaru, Gangwa, Gaourai* (Sanskrit), *Thillai, Akati, Akkolli, Ampala-virutcham, Ampalatti, Kokkumeni, Varivanam, Atiya-kuttam, Paruvi* (Tamil).

Botanical Description: A small mangrove tree to 3-10 m in height with large amount of white latex, bark grayish, leaves alternate, elliptic-obovate. Flowers unisexual, male flowers in catkin spikes, fragrant, yellow, 2.1-3.2 mm across, Stamens 3, filament free. Female flowers in axillary raceme, pale green, 2.6-3.6 mm across, pedicellate, calyx-3-lobed, ovary-3-celled, fruits capsule, globose 3-lobed, seeds sub-globose.

Flowering and Fruiting: Throughout the year

Distribution: India, Philippines, Bangladesh, Australia, Sri Lanka, China, Taiwan, Thailand, Africa, Malaysia, Southern Japan and Pacific Islands.

Propagation: By seeds.

Parts Used: Leaves, latex, bark, fruits and roots

Phytochemical Constituents: The plant contains piperidine alkaloid, phorbol esters, Agallochins A-E, Agallochols A and B, diterpenoids, triterpenoids, flavonoid, phorbole esters, flavanone glycoside, phenols, tannins, terpenoids, glycosides, polyphenols.

Medicinal Uses: The plant is used for leprosy, toothache, epilepsy, dermatitis, conjunctivitis, paralysis and rheumatism. It is also a drastic purgative, abortifacient, antifungal, antimicrobial, antioxidant, anticancer, antitumor and anti-ulcer agent. They are used for treating skin diseases, abdominal troubles, elephantiasis, snake bites, sores, ulcers, diarrhoea, oils and haemorrhages.

Poisonous Parts: Latex

Toxic Constituents: Phorbol esters

Poisonous Symptoms: White latex is injurious to eyes, as it causes rapid blistering and temporary blindness due to contact. The latex is excessively poisonous. The poisonous sap can cause dangerous inflammation of the eyes. Even the smoke of burning wood of this plant is caustic and can cause severe irritation to the eyes.

Gloriosa Superba L.
Family: Colchicaceae

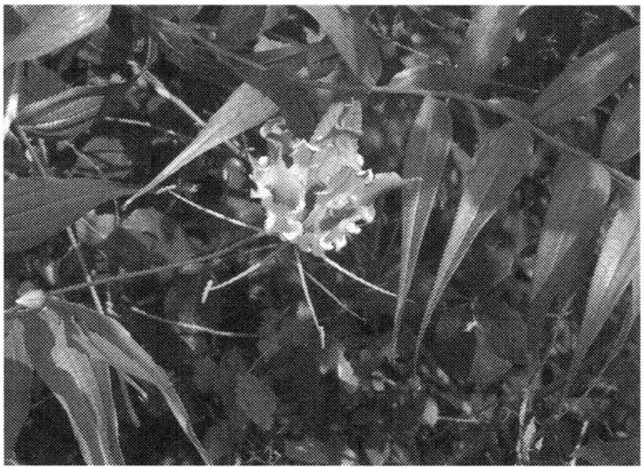

Vernacular Names: *Kannuvalikodi, Kalappaikizhangu* (Tamil), *Nabhi,Gloriosa, Adaviabhi* (Telugu), *Kandal, Kithonni* (Malayalam), *Flamelily, Climbing lily* (English), *Agnimukhi, Agnijvala* (Sanskrit), *Kalihari, Carrihari* (Hindi), *Akkatangaballi, Aginsikhe* (Kannada).

Botanical Description: An annual climbing perennial herb with tuberous roots, rootstock a horizontal rhizome, 3.5 to 6 m in length. Weak stemmed, leaves alternate, rarely opposite or in whorled, lanceolate, sessile 6. 13.5 x 1-3.8 cm, base heart-shaped, apex modified into tendrils which are highly coiled, margin entire, hairless, flowers 7-12 cm across, bisexual, solitary or may form a lax subcorymbose inflorescence, twisted and crisped with six recurved or relexed petals. Blossoming yellow and changing to yellow red and deep scarlet. Stamens 6, spreading, filaments 3.8 x 4.7 cm. Ovary oblong, 3-celled, capsule ellipsoidal, many seeds.

Flowering and Fruiting: August-December.

Distribution: Throughout India.

Propagation: By seeds and tubers.

Parts Used: Roots, leaves and flowers

Phytochemical Constituents: The plant contains colchicine, silosterol, glucoside, beta and Gamma lumicolichicines. Beta silosterol, flucoside, 2-H-6-MeO benzoic acid. Luteolin, glucoside, N-Formyl-de-Me-colchicine, its glucoside and 2-de-Me-colchicine. Benzoic, salicylic acid, sterols and resinous. Substances - colchicines, 3-demethyl colchicine, 1,2-didemethyl colchicine, 2,3-didemethyl colchicine, N-formyl, N-deacetyl colchicines, colchicocide, gloriosine, tannins and superbine. B.sitosterol, chelidonic acid, luteolin and stigmasterol etc.

Medicinal Uses: Root tuber is anthelmintic, purgative and used to treat leprosy. It is also used in piles and skin diseases. Leaves are used to demolish head lice. Roots are purgative, anthelmintic, antiperiodic, cholagogue, astringent, germicidal. It is also used to cure leprosy, swelling, piles, chronic ulcers, colic pain in bladder. Tubers are tonic and anthelmintic and abortifacient. Tubers paste is applied externally and is used as antidote in snake bite. Root powder is given for treatment of rheumatic fever. The plants are used in treating sores, tumours, syphilis and spleen complaints. It exhibits anti-inflammatory, antithrombotic, anticoagulant, enzyme inhibitory, analgesic, antivenom, chemotherapeutic and anticancer properties. All parts of the plant are medicinal and possess antimicrobial properties, antipoxviral potential, larvicidal, skin diseases and respiratory disorders. The root is used as a germicide, to treat ulcers, piles, haemorrhoids, inflammation, scrofula, leprosy, dyspepsia, flatulence, intermittent fever, debility, arthritis and snake poison. The leaves are used in snake bite. Leaves are given to cattle for antiworm treatment. Decoction of the tuber is taken internally to treat aphrodisiac. 50 ml of the tuber juice is mixed with Cow's milk and taken orally to treat piles, gonorrhoea and leprosy.

Poisonous Parts: Roots and tubers

Toxic Constituents: Colchicine, superbine, glucosine and gloriosine

Poisonous Symptoms: Tuber decoction mixed with sugar is used as abortifacient. Intake of the tuber causes vomiting, respiratory poison and may even lead to death. Single tuber is enough to kill human being.

Jatropha Curcas L.

Family: Euphorbiaceae

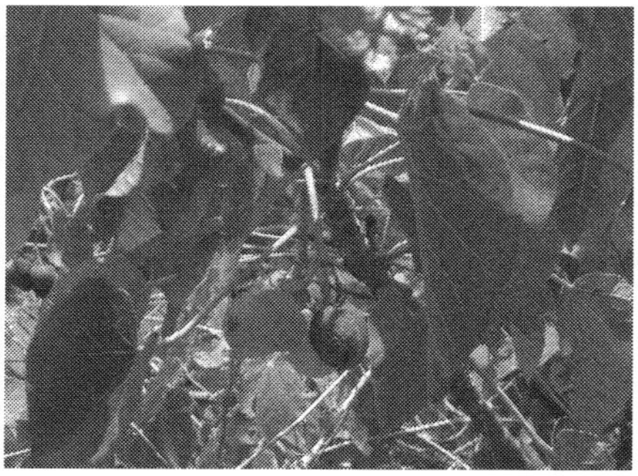

Vernacular Names: *Purging nut, Physic nut* (English), *Errand, Paharierrand, Ratanjot* (Hindi), *Katalavanakku, Kammotti, Kattavanakku* (Malayalam), *Nepalamu, Amudamu* (Telugu), *Danti, Kaattukkottai, Kattamanakku, Katalamanakku* (Tamil), *Bagbherenda, Erandagachh* (Bengali), *Ratanjota, Jamalgota* (Gujarati), *Jahazigaba* (Odisha), *Bongalibhotora* (Assam).

Botanical Description: Large shrub grows up to 3-6 m in height with sticky juice, leaves entire, alternate, largely ovate, shallowly 5-lobed, cordate, 7-17 x 6.145 cm, glabrous base 5-nerved, petiole 5.8-16.3 cm, stipules zero. Cymes to 14 cm; bracts lanceolate, 1.7 cm flowers ca. 8.3 mm across. Stamens 10, anthers 1.6 mm, fruits are 2.6 cm, long ovoid, black, seeds are ovoid-oblong, dull brownish black. The seed resembles castor seed in shape but are smaller in size and dark brown in colour.

Flowering and Fruiting: July - April

Distribution: Throughout India, Indonesia, Malaysia, Mexico, Pakistan and USA.

Propagation: By seeds budding, grafting, air layering

Parts Used: Leaves, latex, seeds, oil bark and stem

Phytochemical Constituents: The fatty acid composition of the oil is as follows; stearic, arachidic, palxitic, myristic linoleic and oleic. The seeds contain curcin, a lectin curcin, raffinose, stachyose, glucose, saccharose, protein and galactose. The plant also contains arachidic, curcasin, stearic and curcin. Aerial part of plant contains coumaric acid, orfanic acid, saponins and tannins. Leaves contain stigmasterol, Stigmastrol-5-en-3, 7 diol, cholest-5-en-3, 7 dil, sitosterol, campesterol, 7-keto - sitosterol, 7-keto-sitoterol. Flavonoids, apigenin, isovitexin, vitexin. Leaves also contain flavonvidal glucoside 30, 31, 32. Latex contain curcacyline A.

Medicinal Uses:

The leaves can serve as rubefacient, galactagogue and insecticide and is useful in treating tumours, scabies, and foul ulcers. The latex is used as purgative, styptic, possesses haemostatic, anti-cancerous properties and is useful in treating ulcers and wounds. The seeds are helpful in treating jaundice and arthritis. The seed can serve as purgative, aphrodisiac, digestive tonic, anthelmintic, depurative and thermogenic agent. It is useful in treating wounds, haemorrhoids and skin diseases. Nuts are used as contraceptives. Latex is used to inhibit watermelon mosaic virus. The stem is used in treating toothache, gum bleeding, gum inflammation and pyorrhoea. Roots act as antidote for snakebite. Oilcake is used as manure.

The oil extracted from seeds shows purgative properties and is used externally in rheumatism. It is also used to cure paralytic affections. Seeds are crushed, and the resulting jatropha oil can be processed to produce a high quality biodiesal or biofuel that can be used in standard diesel. The whole plant is used as rodent repellent and organic fertilizer. The kernels are used for seed cake. It is used in the treatment of dropsy, paralysis, diarrohea, rheumatism, dysentery and several skin diseases. Plant decoction is used in the treatment of burns, cuts, allergies, wound inflammation, leprosy, small pox, leucoderma, and wound healing. Water extract of branches are used to cure HIV and tumor.

Poisonous Parts: Leaves, seeds, bark and latex.

Toxic Constituents: Phorbol esters, which are toxic to humans and animals, trypsin inhibitors phytates, lectin.

Poisonous Symptoms: Latex is injurious to eyes. Leaves and seeds are purgative. If consumed by livestock or human beings particularly children, it causes burning sensation in stomach and vomiting. Over-consumption of seeds leads to unconsciousness. Bark is used as fish poison. The plant is toxic to human beings, causing vomiting, convulsions, diarrhoea, nausea, high pulse, muscle shock, delirium, burning and pain in throat and mouth, leading to death. The plant is toxic to livestock, causing diarrhoea, salivation, dehydration, gastrointestinal inflammation, tumor formation, depression, loss of weight, lack of appetite, reduced water intake, hemorrhagic effect in various organs and death. Intake of 5-10 seeds is fatal to adults. Large consumption of seeds by pregnant livestock causes abortion.

Jatropha Gossypifolia L.
Family: Euphorbiaceae

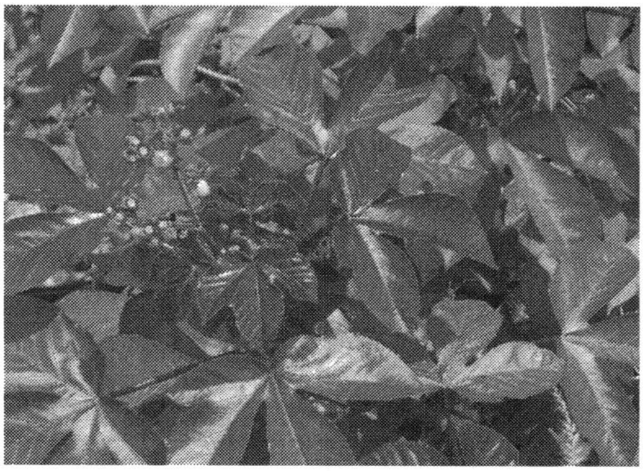

Vernacular Names: *Cotton leaf, Puppet seed plant* (English), *Ratanjoti* (Hindi), *Lal Bharenda* (Bengali), *Chikka kada maralu* (Kannada), *E-hidak* (Manipuri), *Seemayavanakku, Chuvanna kadalavanakku* (Malayalam), *Siria Amanakku, Athalai* (Tamil), *Ratanjyot* (Gujarat).

Botanical Description: Grows to 2.8-5 m. The three lobed leaves are purple and sticky when young and becomes bright green with age. Leaves dark green, alternate, simple ovate to slightly lobed with 3-5, upto 15.2 cm wide, flowers yellow to green in colour. Capsule 2.7-4.1 cm. These are green and fleshy when immature, becoming dark brown when ripe spitting to release 2-3 black seeds. Seeds oblong, trigonous.

Flowering and Fruiting: Throughout the year

Distribution: Australia, Mexico, South America, Caribbean Islands, India, Malaysia, China, Indonesia and Philippines

Propagation: By seeds and stem cuttings

Parts Used: Roots, latex, stem, leaves, seeds and fruits

Phytochemical Constituents: Gossypidien, gossypifan, jatrodien, jatrophatrione, jatrophenone, jatropholone A, jatropholone B, Jatrophone, cyclogossine A, cyclogossine B, Isogadain, hydroxyjatrophone, hydroxyiso, jatrophone, terpenoids, flavonoids, tannins, alkaloids, cardiac glycosides, saponin.

Medicinal Uses: The seeds are purgative, abortifacient, anthelminthic, and are used to treat skin disorders and paralysis. The seed oil is used to treat itching, rheumatic conditions, parasitic skin ailments and in the curing of jaundice, fever, gonorrhoea, eczema, constipation, leprosy, and is used as a diuretic and mouth wash. The leaf is used as haemostatic, antimicrobial, anti-inflammatory agent. The bark is used as a fish poison, and can exhibit antifeedant activity, antidiabetic activity, hypolipidemic activity. The main use is as renewable source of energy as biodiesel. The leaf decoction is used for bathing wounds, fever. The young stem and latex with foetid smell is used as toothbrush, and cures mouth ulcer.

Poisonous Part: Leaves, latex seeds and seed pods.

Toxic Constituents: Curcin a phytotoxin, ricinoleic acid, crotonoleic acid and hydrocyaic acid.

Poisonous Symptoms: Leaves and seeds are potent purgative and poisonous. Latex is injurious to eyes, cause blindness. If consumed by cattle, causes severe vomiting followed by death symptoms and are broadly these associated with gastro-intestinal irritation, abdominal pain, burning sensation, nausea, vomiting and diarrhoea.

Lantana Camara L.

Family: Verbenaceae

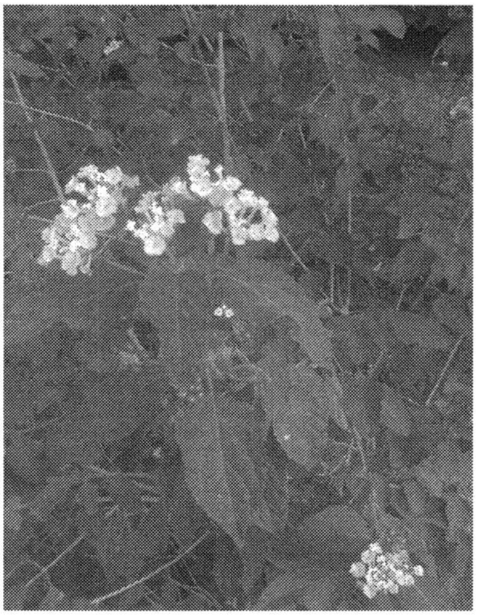

Vernacular Names: *Lantana weed, Wild sage* (English), *Lantana, Bunch berry, Caturang, Ghaneri* (Hindi),*Caturangi, Vanacchedi, Jhingini* (Sanskrit), *Unnichti, Arippu, Arisimalar* (Tamil), *Pulikampa, Akshinte Poolu* (Telugu), *Arippu, Pucceti* (Malayalam), *Lantavanigidda, Kadugulabi* (Kannada), *Thirei, Nongballei, Samballei* (Manipuri).

Botanical Description: Large scrambling evergreen, strong smelling shrub with stont recurved prickles and a strong odour of black currents. Plant grows up to 1 to 4 meters and it can spread to

3 meter in width. Leaves are ovate or ovate oblong, acute-sub acute, crenate serrate, rugore above, scabrid on both sides. The leaves are 3-9 cm long by 3-7 cm wide and green in colour. Leaves and stem are covered with rough hairs, small flower held in clusters. Colour commonly, orange, sometime varying from red or white in several shades and the flower generally change colours as they ages, flowers are having a yellow throat, in axillary head. The calyx is small corolla tube slender. Stamens 4 in two pairs. Fruits 0.5-0.7 cm across, fleshy drupes, 6mm in diameter, endocarp hard grey when young and blue or black on ripening.

Flowering and Fruiting: Throughout the year.

Distribution: Native of USA, runs wild throughout India, both in the plains and hills. Australia, Brazil, Indonesia, Kenya, Uganda, Tanzania, Pakistan, Mexico, Jamaica, Africa, Caribbean and New Zealand

Propagation: By seeds and stem cuttings

Parts Used: Entire parts of the plant.

Phytochemical Constituents: The plant contains alkaloids, steroids, saponins, triterpenes, tannin, glycosides, iridoid, phonye ethanoid, phenolic compounds, flavonoids, carbohydrates and proteins. Tannare, invertase, amylase, catalase, and glucosidase. Appreciable amounts of sugar and tannins, crystalline glucoside have been separated from the resin by ether extraction.

Caryophyllene lantadene A, lantadene B which is inactive and a steroid, lantanine, lancamarone quinine, like alkaloid.

Medicinal Uses: The plant exhibits antipyretic, carminative, antiseptic, antispasmodic, anti-inflammatory analgesic and diaphoretic properties. It is also used in exhibiting antibacterial activity, antifungal activity, wound healing activity, anti-inflammatory activity, hemolytic activity, anticancer activity, anti-filarial activity, mosquito controlling activity, anthelmintic, hepatoprotective activity, antioxidant activity, larvicidal activity, anticancer activity.

Leaves are used to cure tetanus, ulcers, cancers, asthma, swelling, eczema, tumor, chicken pox, cuts, rheumatisms, catarrhal infection, high blood pressure, measles, fevers, ataxy of abdominal viscera, sores, cold and high blood pressure. The whole plant is used to treat bronchitis and the root is powdered and mixed with milk and is given to children for stomachache and as a vermifuge. Lantana oil is used to manage skin diseases, itches, and as an antiseptic for wounds. Root decoction is used in treating dysentery. Leaf powder is used in treating ulcers, wounds and cuts. The fruits are used for treatment of rheumatism and tumours.

Poisonous Parts: Entire plant, especially the berries and fruits.

Toxic Constituents: Lantanine, lancamarone, lantadenes A, lantadenes B, polycyclic terpenoid lantadene, lantadene C and lantadene D.

Poisonous Symptoms: Grazing of animals cause severe injury to liver, loss of appetite, weakness, failure of blood circulation, profuse salivation, copious lachrymation, diarrhoea, gastro intestinal irritation with abdominal pain and death in severe condition. Jaundice and some degree of photosensitivity may occur. Unripe berries are toxic to humans, causing vomiting, labored respiration, weakness and diarrhea.

Melia Azedarach L.

Family : Meliaceae

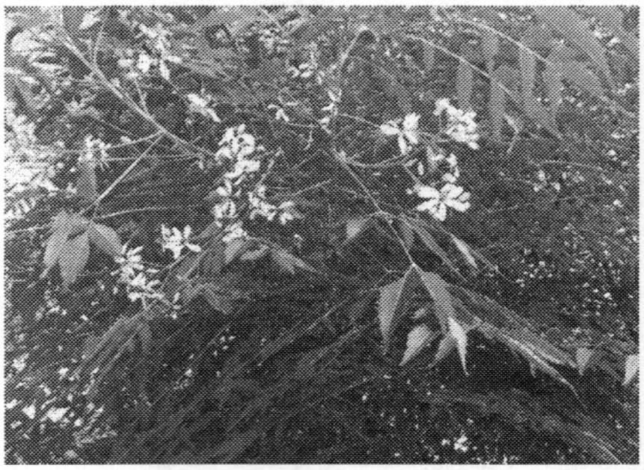

Vernacular Names: *China berry, Morgosa tree, pride of India, umbrella tree, bead tree, Indian liliac* (English), *Arista, Mahanimba, Akshadru* (Sanskrit), *Kattu vembu, Malaivembu, Malaiveppam* (Tamil), *Drek, Bakain, Bakarja* (Hindi), *Konda-vepa, Koda-vepa* (Telugu), *Karin vembu, Arya veppu, Malaveppu* (Malayalam), *Arebevu, Bettada-berina* (Kannada), *Mahanim, ghora nim* (Bengali).

Botanical Description: A tree, 5-15 m height or more, bark grey, greyish brown, lenticellate, rectangular scaly in old trees. Leaves bi or tri-pennate, 25-75 cm long. Leaflets 2.8-5.2 x 1.2-2.6 cm, leaflets opposite, serrate, glabrous on both sides. Inflorescence in terminal biparous cyme or axillary. Flowers 1.2-1.6 cm across, white-lilac, drupe ovate or ellipsoid-globose, yellow when ripe, 4 to 5 black seeds.

Flowering and Fruiting: July - December

Distribution: Native to India, China, Africa, Australia, USA and Argentina

Propagation: By seeds and vegetative method

Parts Used: Bark, flowers, leaf, roots and seeds.

Phytochemical Constituents: The plant contains arginine, glycine, cystine, lycine, bakayanin, rutin, methionine, leucine, threonine, serine, proline, quercitrin, backalactone 6 β-hydroxy-4-stigmastem-3-one and 6 β-hydroxy-4-cappesten-3-one, 4,5-dihydroxy-7-O-γ-L-rhamnopyranosyl-(1→74)-β-D-glucopyranoside and glutamic acid. The leaves contain the flavonoid rutin and the alkaloid paraisine. The root bark and stem bark contain tannins, alkaloid azaridine and sterols. The seeds yield the oleic, linoleic acids, stearic and palmitic.

Medicinal Uses: The leaf paste is applied externally to treat skin ailments, leprosy and nervous disorders. The flowers are powdered and mixed with Cow's milk and is given orally for headache. It can serve as an antifeedant and insecticide. The leaves are used as diuretic, resolvent, deobstruent, antibacterial, anthelmintic agent. The leaves can be used to treat small pox, viral fever, skin infections, leprosy and scrofula. Seed oil is used as antiseptic for sores and ulcers. It is also used in treating skin ailments, rheumatism, ringworm and scabies. The seed oil mixed with sugar is given orally for malaria fever and leprosy. Fresh leaf decoction is applied externally for burns. Fresh leaf juice is used as mouth wash. Leaf decoction 10 ml is administered orally twice a day for two days to cure piles. Leaf juice 5-10 ml is administered orally thrice a day for 5 days to treat pyrexia. Stem bark exhibits antiviral, anticancerous and antispasmodic activity. The bark decoction is given to control women hormone sickness and is also an antiseptic.

Poisonous Parts: Seeds and leaves

Toxic Constituents: Alkaloids and tannins

Poisonous Symptoms: Leaves are poisonous, used as insecticide. Intake of seeds causes nausea, acute irritation and degeneration of the kidney and liver.

Momordica Charantia L.

Family: Cucurbitaceae

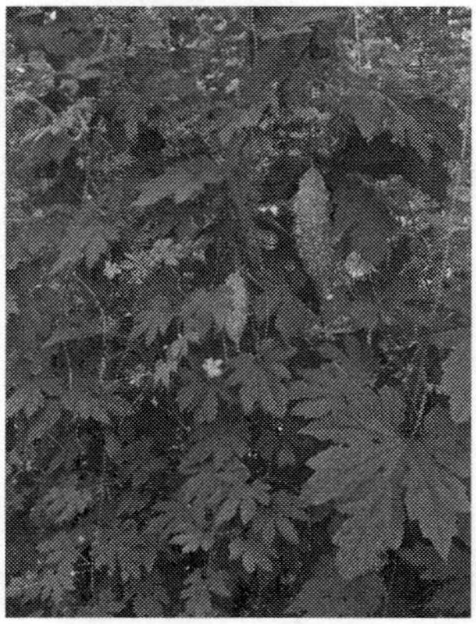

Vernacular Names: *Balsam apple, Bitter Melon, Bitter guard, Balsam pear* (English), *Karala* (Bengali), *Karelu* (Gujarati), *Karela* (Assamese), *Kathilla, Poraru, Karela* (Hindi), *Haagalakaay* (Kannada), *Kaaraate* (Malayalam), *Karon akhabi* (Manipuri), *Changkha* (Marathi), *Urdhvaasitah* (Odisa), *Paaharkaai* (Tamil), *Kaarvellakah, Kathillah, Paraaru, Sushavi* (Sanskrit), *Kakara* (Telugu).

Botanical Description: An herbaceous climber, much branched angled stems, leaves simple, unusally palmate, 5-9 lobed, tendrils 2 branched or unbranched, tendril bearing vine grows to 4.6m. Staminate flowers normally solitary on a bracteate scape, hypanthium shallow, calyx 5 lobed, petals 5 normally yellow distinct, 1-3 with incurved scales at base, stamnes 3, anthers distinct ovules several horizontal, stigmas 3, 2 lobed fruit 2.7 - 20 cm, ovoid, ellipsoid or spindle shaped many immersed in bright red pulp, ovate, commonly sculptured. Each plant produces different yellow female and male flowers.

Flowering and Fruiting: Throughout the year

Distribution: Asia, Australia, Tropical Africa, India, China, East Africa, South America, Amazon, Caribbean, Bangladesh, Cuba, Brazil, Malaysia, Panama, Peru, Nicaragua and Nigeria.

Propagation: By seeds.

Parts Used: Leaves, root fruit and seeds

Phytochemical Constituents: The seeds contain alkaloids, steroids, flavonoids, glycosides oil, fats, phenols, tannins, amino acids, valine, leucine, isoleucine, methionine, threonine glutamic acid and phenylalanine. The leaves, fruits and seeds include α and β - monorcharin.

The plant contains various biologically active compounds mainly momordicin I and momordicin II and cucurbitacin B. The plant also contains many bioactive glycosides including momordicosides, charanin, momordin, charantosides, goyaglycosides, and other terpeniod compounds including momordicilin, momordenoil, momordicinin, momordicin-28 and momordol. It also contains momorcharin and momordin. The fruit contains alkaloids resins, saponins, momordicine, charantin, alanine, serine, glutamic acid, itreonine, phenolic constituents, glycosides, fixed oil, free acids and reducing sugar. The leaves of the plant have been found to contain alkaloid, sterols, terpenoids, flavonoids, phenols, proteins and anthroquinones.

Several biochemical constituents namely cucurbitins, cucurbitanes, cucurbitacins, momordicosides, momordenol, momordicines, momorcharins, momordin, momordicinin, momordicilin, charantin, alkaloids, charine, oxalic sacid, oleics acid, proteins, lanosterol, karounidiols, Olanolic acid, steroidal glycosides, cryptoxanthin and erythrodiol have been isolated from various parts of the plant. They are uracil, vacine, vicine, taraxerol, spinasterol, rubixanthin. V-insulin, verbascoside, amino acids - aspartic acid, serine, glutamic acid, lycopene, pipecolic acid, alanine, b-sitosterol-d-glucoside, g-amino butyric acid, multiflorenol and myristic acid are also present.

Medicinal Uses:

The plant is antidiabetic, antibacterial, antifungal, antimicrobial, antioxidant, antitumor, anti-inflammatory, antimycobacterial, antiulcer and aphrodisiac. It is used for its cytotoxic, anthelmintic, antibiotic, anti mutagenic, antiviral, hormonal, antileukemic, tonic, insecticidal, stomachic, laxative, vermifuge, styptic, refrigerant and purgative properties. It is also useful as laxative, hypotensive, carminative, hypoglycemic, refrigerant and immunostimulant.

The root is used to treat diabetes, dyspepsia, constipation, malaria, cancer, asthma, snake bite, fever, anemia, hepatitis and insecticide. They are useful to treat stomachache, cough, hypertension, gonorrhea, dysentery, leprosy, digestion, burn, catarrh, headache, pneumonia, rheumatism and kidney stone. It is used to cure eczema, emetic, dermatosis, rheumatoid arthritis. It can act as vermifuge, aphrodisiac, astringent and abortifacient and is known for its wound healing activity, larvicidal activity and menstrual colic.

The fruit is considered as stomachic, tonic, stimulant, emetic, laxative, antibilous alterative. The fruit is used to treat diabetes, dyspepsia, constipation, liver diseases, rheumatism, goat and subacute cases of the spleen. The fruit juice or leaf tea treats malaria, diabetes, sores and wounds, colic infections, worms and parasites, hepatitis, fever. Leaf juice, fruit pulp and seeds exhibit anthelmintic properties. Leaves are used as galactogogue. Immature fruit is employed for treating cancer, malaria and possess antiviral properties, anti HIV properties.

Poisonous Parts: Juice of plant, outer fruit coat, seed and ripe fruit.

Toxic Constituents: Alkaloids, resin and saponic glycosides and vicine.

Poisonous Symptoms: Excessive consumption of seed, ripe fruit, fruit coat and plant juice causes diarrhea, cathartic and produces gastroenteritis with vomiting, headache, muscular weakness, salivation, facial redness, stomach pain, nausea, pupil dilation. Toxic only if enormous quantities are eaten.

Moringa Oleifera Lam.

Family: Moringaceae

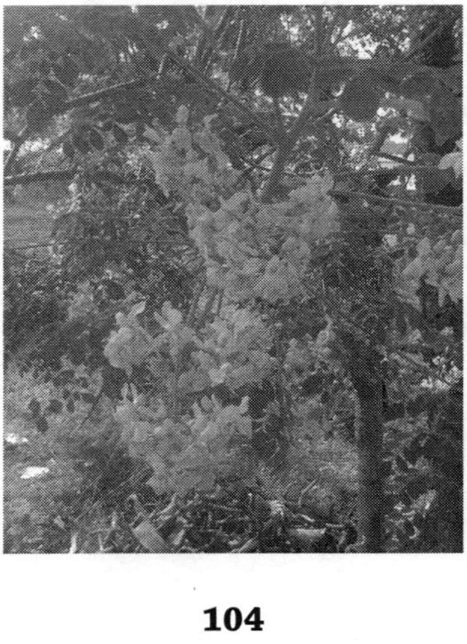

Vernacular Names: *Horseradish tree, Drum stick tree* (English), *Danshamula, Sobanjana* (Sanskrit), *Murunkai - kai, Murungai, Morunga* (Tamil), *Moringa, Sigru, Muringa* (Malayalam), *Tella - Munaga, Munaga, Sajna, Sojna* (Bengali), *Saragavo, Midho - Saragavo* (Gujarathi), *Munigha, Sajina* (Odisha), *Murunga, Nuggi* (Kannada), *Mungana, Sahijan* (Hindi).

Botanical Description: Short, deciduous, slender, perennial tree, growing to about 10 m tall, with corky bark and soft white wood. Leaves feathery, pale green, alternate, 3-5-pinnate, 30-60 cm long. There are 2-9 leaflets on the ultimate pinnules. Leaflets are thin, ovate to elliptic and 1-2cm long. Flowers fragrant white or creamy - white 2.5 cm in diameter, 2 cm long 5 merous, stamens yellow. The pod is 12-40 cm long. Pendulous, three angled and has nine ribs. Seeds light or dark brown, sub-globase, 1.1-1.5 cm diameter with 3 papery wings.

Flowering and Fruiting: Throughout the year.

Distribution: Bangladesh, Malaysia, Nepal, Pakistan, Cambodia, Sri Lanka, India, Indonesia, Tropical Africa, Caribbean Islands, Nigeria, Thailand, Vietnam and Philippines.

Propagation: By seeds and cuttings

Parts Used: Leaves, flowers, fruit and seed

Phytochemical Constituents: The plant contains upiol, adenine, palmitic acid, linalool oxide. The leaves contain flavonoids pigments such as rhamnatin, kaempferol, Kaempferitrin and isoquercitrin.

The flowers contain traces of alkaloids. The vital amino acids present in the total proteins are lysine, methionine, leucine, valine, isoleucine, histidine, and arginine. The root contains tannins, carbohydrate, saponins, steroids, flavonoids, alkaloids, cardiac glycosides, pterygospermin. The root bark contains two alkaloids, viz., moringinial and moringine. The plant provides a high and rare combination of β-sitosterol, kaempferol, zeatin, quercetin and caffeoylquinic acid.

Medicinal Uses: The leaves are useful in treating tumours, wounds, anodyne, Scurvy. The leaves are anthelimintic, anti -inflammatory and are high in vitamins A and C. They are used in treating paralysis, fever, diarrhoea and colic flatulence. It is also used as anticancer, anti-ulcer, diuretic, anthelmintic, antioxidant, hepatoprotective, antiurolithiatic, antimicrobial, anti-inflammatory agent. Many parts of this plant namely, leaves, seed, fruit, flowers and young pods act as antipyretic, antihypertensive, antiepileptic, cardiac and circulatory stimulants, control antitumour, antispasmodic, antidiabetic, cholesterol lowering, antifungal, antibacterial, antifertility, antitubercular, abortifacient and as cardiotonic and anti-hypercholesterolaemic agent.

The seed oil serves as antibacterial, antifungal, antiepileptic, anti-inflammatory agent. It is utilized for curing rheumatism, gout and venomous bites. It is also used in all kinds of soap and cosmetic products.

Poisonous Parts: Root bark and stem bark.

Toxic Constituents: Steroids, alkaloids, tannins and saponins.

Poisonous Symptoms: Intake of root bark juice causes acute skin inflammation and skin dermatitis. Stem bark and root bark are utilized as abortifacient.

Mucuna Pruriens (L) DC

Family : Fabaceae

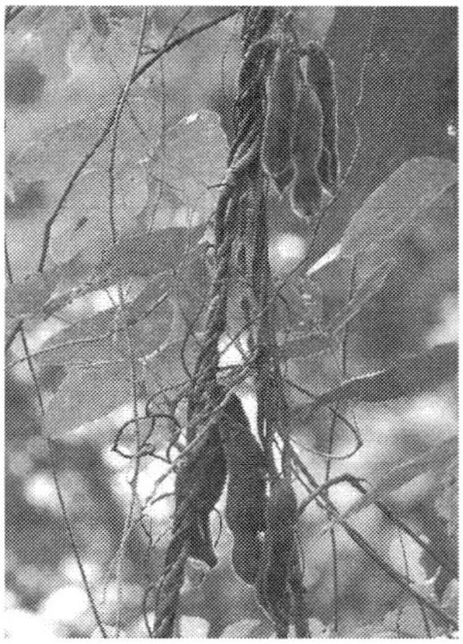

Vernacular Names: Cowhage, Common cowitch (English), Kivacc, Kaunc, Konch, Gonca (Hindi), *Kapikacchuh, Atmagupta* (Sanskrit), *Naykkorana,* corivalli *(Malayalam), Punaippidukkan, Poonaikkali, Punaikali* (Tamil), *Nasuganni, Nasagunnikaayi* (Kannada), *Pilliadugu, Duradagondi* (Telugu), *Alkushil* (Bengali), *Khaajkuiri* (Marathi), *Baidanka* (Odisha).

Botanical Description: An annual, climbing shrub with hairy branches. Leaves are fairly large, alternate, stipulate, pinnately trifoliate, ovate, reverse ovate, racemes 11-25 cm long, flowers dark purple, in axillary pendulous, calyx bilipped, grey, corolla dark - purplish. The fruit contains four to six or more seeds with septa or partitions between the seeds. The seeds are black in colour, reniform in shape, 16-21mm long and 7.16 mm broad, pods oblong, ribbed 4-6 seeded.

Flowering and Fruiting: December - March

Distribution: Throughout India, Sri Lanka, Bangladesh, Malaysia and South East Asia

Propagation: By seeds

Parts Used: Roots, leaves and seeds

Phytochemical Constituents: The seeds contain alkaloids, flavonoids, steroids, phenols, glycosides, protein, tannins, proten, resins, saponins, triterpenoids.

Medicinal Uses: The plant is used to treat diabetes, cancer, cholera, cough, diuretic, edema, dysentery, impotency, menstrual problems, kidney stones, snake bite, scorpion sting, worms, tuberculosis, sterility, and as an aphrodisiac and uterine stimulant. The plant is also used to treat asthma, burns, cuts, dog bite, insanity, mumps, nerves, pain, pleurisy, paralysis, sores, tumors, syphilis, ringworm and as an aphrodisiac, antimicrobial, antioxidant, antibacterial. The seed is used to manage various free radical mediated ailments, rheumatoid arthritis, diabetes, nervous disorders, and can serve as antipyretic and analgesic agent. The roots, leaves and seeds of the plant are used in the treatment of cancer, and diabetes mellitus. The pods is used as anthelmintic and seeds exhibit aphrodisiac and anti-inflammatory properties.

Poisonous Parts: Pods, flowers, bean and seeds.

Toxic Constituents: Steroids, alkaloids and glycosides.

Poisonous Symptoms: Contact with the pod hairs causes the skin itching and sometimes causes blister, dermatitis and blindness if in the eyes.

Nerium Oleander L.

Family: Apocynaceae

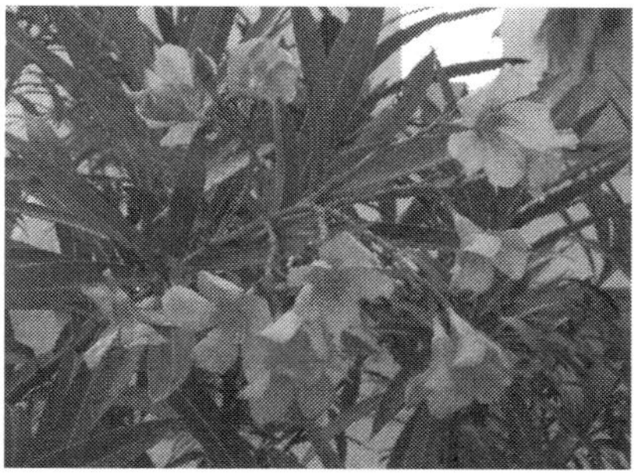

Vernacular Names: *Indian oleander, Sweet scanted oleander* (English),*Karavirah, Asvahana* (Sanskrit), *Chandni, Kanir, Karber, Kaner, Karuvira* (Hindi), *Sevvarali, Arali, Alari, Irattai, Sivapparai* (Tamil),*Arali, Kanaviram, Karaviram* (Malayalam), *Kanagailu, Dhavekaneri, Paddale, Chandaatha* (Kannada), *Erra ganneru, Karavivamu Ganneru, Kasthuripatti* (Telugu).

Botanical Description: Grows to 3-8m wide glabrous evergreen shrub with latex, leaves are 10-25cm long, normally ternate, shortly stalked, linear, lanceolate, glossy, green above, nerves, obscure, several, parallel; flowers white, red and rose coloured in terminal cymes; The fruit consists of a long narrow capsule 10 to 13 cm long and 6.5 to 8.3 mm in diameter.

Flowering and Fruiting: Throughout the year

Distribution: Afghanistan, Nepal, Japan and cultivated throughout India

Propagation: By stem cuttings

Parts Used: Roots and leaves

Phytochemical Constituents: Whole parts of the plant are toxic substances. Root, bark and seeds contain neriodorein, karabin, cardio-active glycosides, earliearly adesignated as neriodorin, neriodorin and karabin were noted tohave in paralyzoing performance on the heart, like digitalin and a stimulating activity on the spinal cord, like strychnine, proteins, alkaloids, flavonoids, terpenoids, tannins, saponins.

Medicinal Uses: The leaves are a potent repellent and are utilized for scabies, haemorhoids. Tender leaves juice is useful for ophthalmia with copious lacrimation. The roots are used in anthelmintic, astringent, stomachic, diuretic and febrifuge. They are useful in treating asthma, renal, leprosy, pruritus, arthralgia, stomachalgia and ulcers. The flowers are reported to have the characteristic of purifying the air. The plant exhibits anti-inflammatory activity, antioxidant, antimicrobial, antitumor, antiabacterial activity, antinociceptive activity.

This plant is proven to exhibit toxicity to human and animals, but it is also proved to contain medicinal value like antibacterial property. The leaves are used in maceration and in external friction, false scabies, hair loss, lice, toothache and diabetes.

Poisonous Parts: All parts especially leaves, stem, seeds and roots

Toxic Constituents: Cardiac glycosides as oleandroside, nerioside, neriodorin, neriodererin, karabin oleandrin and nerine.

Poisonous Symptoms: Whole parts of the plant are poisonous. Root and root bark are poisonous, causes cardiac poison, used for criminal and suicidal purposes. Seeds are used as poison to kill animals. Leaves, stem and roots causes drowsiness, increased pulse rate, abdominal pain, vomiting, gastroenteritis with dizziness, and other miscellaneous symptoms are followed by breathing difficulties, an irregular and weakened heart beat, coma and eventually death.

Severe diarrhea, abdominal pain, sweating and weakness are the common symptoms. These signs appear within few hours after eating the leaves. Consumption of flowers causes nausea to humans. Intake of leaves by animals results in vomiting, abdominal pain, weakness, bloody diarrhoea for one or three days.

Nicotiana Tabacum L.

Family: Solanaceae

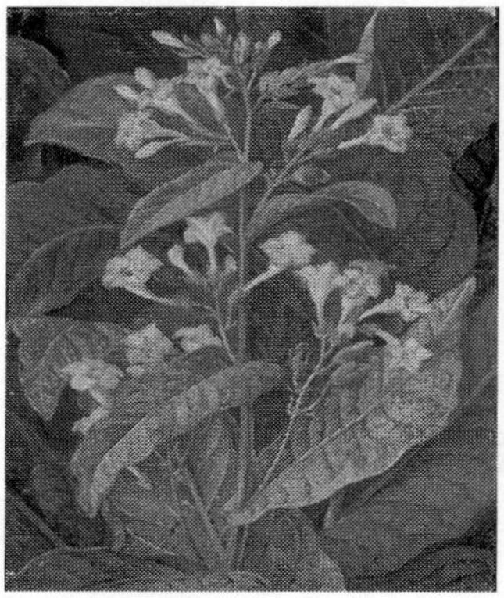

Vernacular Names: *Tobacco* (English), *Tobacco, Tamaku, Tampaku, Bujjerbhang* (Hindi), *Dhumrapatra, Tamakhuh* (Sanskrit), *Pugaiyilai* (Tamil), *Pogaku, Dhumrapatramu* (Telugu), *Pukayila, Pokala* (Malayalam), *Tambaku, Hogesoppu* (Kannada)

Botanical Description: Erect, glandular pubescent herb few branches, leaves broad oblong or elliptic - ovate 26-60 x 24-50 cm, base largely acute, upper leaves narrowed, lanceolate; flowers light red, white or pink in several flowers panicled recemes; calyx 1.2cm; lobes 5, corolla rose, 1.6 cm across; stamens 5, attached at the same level. Ovary 4.2 mm; style 5.2 cm, fruits narrowly elliptic, ovoid capsule; seeds several, brown with fluted ridges.

Flowering and Fruiting: August - March

Distribution: USA, Argentina, Brazil, India, Cuba, Ecuador, Guatemala, Iran, Mexico, Canada, Tanzania, East Africa and Sri Lanka.

Propagation: By seeds and vegetative technique.

Parts Used: Leaves.

Phytochemical Constituents: Nicotimine, nornicotine, nictyrine, anabasine, nicotimine, nicotelline, myosamine, Nicotoine, Piperidine, Pyrrolidine, glucosides, 2,3,6-trimethyl-1, 4-naphthoquinone, 2-methylquinone, 2-napthylamine, propionic acid, anatlline, anthalin, acrolein, anethole, anatabine, cembrene, choline and pyrene.

Medicinal Uses: The leaves are beneficial as narcotic, sedative, anodyne, laxative, styptic, mental stimulant, anti-inflammatory, abortifacient and anthelmintic agent. They are used in dental caries, inflammations, dyspepsia, flatulence, bronchitis, asthma, skin ailments, scabies, painful tumours, helminthiasis and purulent discharge from the nose. The nicotine of tobacco is used as an insecticide, Instillation of tobacco enemal for treatment of constipation. The plant is used in antimicrobial activity.

Poisonous Parts: Whole parts except ripe seeds.

Toxic Constituents: Nicotine and other alkaloids, anabasine and anatabine.

Poisonous Symptoms: Consumption of leaves causes vomiting, slow pulse, diarrhea, collapse, dizziness and respiratory failure. At low doses, it causes nausea, vomiting, diarrhoea, salivation and dizziness. At higher doses, abdominal pain marked with severe diarrhoea and cold sweat mental confusion, giddiness, restlessness, muscular weakness and disturbed vision and unconsciousness. Respiration is stimulated, pulse is rapid and irregular and breathing is laboured. It causes cardiac arrest and respiratory paralysis.

Oxalis Corniculata L.

Family: Oxalidaceae

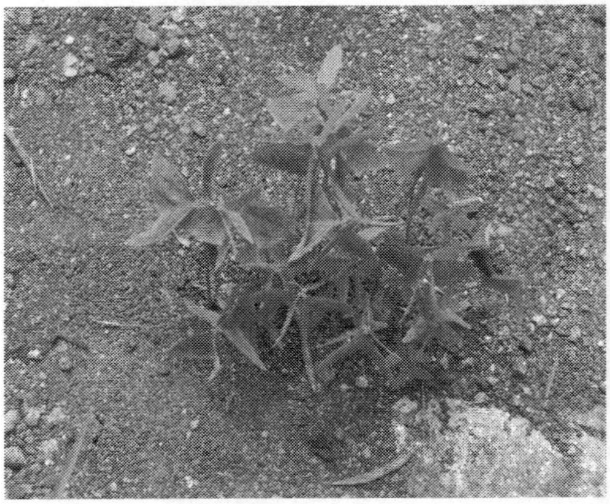

Vernacular Names: *Yellow sorrel, Indian sorrel, Creeping wood sorrel, Creeping oxalis, Wood Sorre* (English), *Amlapatrika, Amilika, Ahangen* (Sanskrit), *Amrulsak, Tinpatiya, Chukkatripati* (Hindi), *Puliyaral, Pullampurachi, Puliyarala* (Malayalam), *Puliyarai, Puliakire, Palaikiri, Puliyarani* (Tamil), *Ambotikura, Pulichintaku* (Telugu), *Hulichikkal, Pullam purachi, Uppinasoppu* (Kannada), *Chukka tripati, Amrui shak* (Bengali), *Yensil* (Manipuri), *Tengecl tenga* (Assamese), *Amboti, Chicha, Ambali* (Marathi), *Khatta sag* (Urdu), *Sialthur, Siakthur, Ambocingari* (Odisha).

Botanical Description: A small creeping perennial herb that forms roots and nodes, leaves alternate, trifoliate, leaflets obcordate. Petiole 2.1-2.7 cm, petiolule 0, Pseudo-umbels axillary. Flowers yellow, 5-merous, calyx 5, ovate, corolla yellow, oblaneolate, 6.1 x 3.2mm. Stamens 10, filaments 2.7 and 3.6 mm. Ovary 5 celled, fruit a sub-cylindrical capsule up to 19 cm long. Containing many tiny black seeds.

Flowering and Fruiting: Throughout the year.

Distribution: India, Naturalized worldwide China, USA, Mexico and West Indies.

Propagation: By seeds

Parts Used: Whole plant.

Phytochemical Constituents: Oxalic acid, Vitexin and isovitexin, glyxylic acid, glycolipids, neutral lipids, vitexin-2-0-beta-d-glucopyranoide, vitamin c, fatty acids, phospholipids, tranphyto, 2-heptenal, 2-pentylfurn, beta-tocopherols and D glucopyranoside. The plant contains tannins, flavonoids, phenol, glycosides, fatty acids, phytosterols, volatile oil and galacto-glycerolipid. The leaves contain flavonoids, vitexine-2''-o-beta-D-glucopyrunoside and isovitexine, oleic, linoleic, palxitic acid, linolenic and stearic acids. The whole plant contains alkaloids, glycosides, fixed oils and fats, carbohydrates, saponins, phenolic compounds, protein, amino acids, gums and mucilage.

Medicinal Uses: The plant is used as a medication for convulsions in children and for healing fractured bones. The plant is used to treat wounds, burns, and body sores. The leaf juice is applied to open wounds. Leaf is astringent, refrigerant, coolant, anti-scorbutic and appetising agent. It is used to treat fever. Leaf pate is applied externally, used as antidote for snake bite. Ground leaves are also utilized in curing diarrhoea, dizziness and dysentery. It is utilized to cure sores and wounds and swelling beneath tongue. The plant is utilized in exhibiting antimicrobial activity, anti-cancer activity, anti-oxidant activity, anti-inflammatory activity, analgesic, steroidogenic, anti-mioebic, antifungal, astringent, diuretic, depurative, febrifuge, cardio relaxant, styptic and stomachic. The plant possess anti-ulcer activity antiseptic and hepatoprotective activity.

Poisonous Parts: Whole plant.

Toxic Constituents: Soluble oxalate.

Poisonous Symptoms: Leaves are poisonous, causes removal of calcium ions in the serum by precipitation, immediate death as an effect of extensive renal injure. Large doses may cause cramps, trembling and staggering as in grazing cattle.

Parthenium Hysterophors L.

Family: Asteraceae

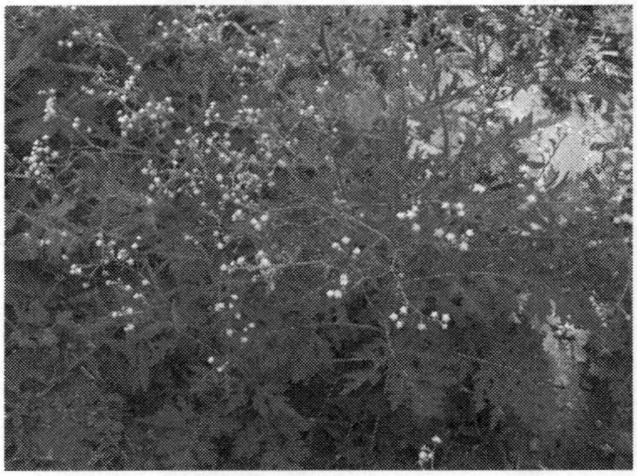

Vernacular Names: *Santa maria fever few, Congress,grass, Congree grass, Carrot grass* (English), *Chatak can dani, Gajar Ghas* (Hindi), *Parthenium* (Tamil), *Coimbatore chedi* (Irula tribes), *Congress Pacha*

Botanical Description: Much branched annual or ephemeral herb plant growing 75 cm to 160 cm height. The leaves are irregularly dissected and pubescent. Leaves are pale green simple alternate, pinnately or bipinnately deeply lobed and covered with fine soft hairs. The stem is hairy octiangular, longitudinally grooved. The stem and leaf surface is covered with four types of glanular and non-glandular multicellular while trichomes, white about 4mm across, arising from the leaf forks enormous number of pollen grains. The fruits are broadly obovoid in shape and have dark brown colour. Seeds 2 mm long. Each flower produces 4 to 5 black wedge shaped seeds.

Flowering and Fruiting: Throughout the year.

Distribution: Native to Mexico, USA, India, Africa, Australia, Asia and Pacific Islands, Caribbean, Jamaica, West Indies, China, Nepal, Vietnam, Brazil and Argentina.

Propagation: By seeds

Parts Used: All parts

Phytochemical Constituents: The plant contains, bitter glycoside parthenin, sesquiterpene lactones, hysterin, ambrosin, flavonoids, caffeic acid, vanillic acid, pcourmaric, anisic acid, p-anisic acid, chlorogenic acid, ferulic acid, and sitosterol. The plant contains a great number of important bioactive compounds, flavonoid, glycosides, pinenes, terpenoids, volatile oils, histamine amino acids, saponins, phenolic derivatives and amino sugars. The leaves contain parthenin, myricylalcohol, hexacosanol, campesterol, betulin, ursolic acid, stigmasterol, β-sitpsterol, β-D-glucoside of β-sitosterol and saponin. The flowers contain parthenin, coronopilin, and hysterone. The roots contain parthenin, caffeic, vailic, salicylic, neo-chlorogenic proto-catechuic acids, p-hydroxybenzoic, p-anisic and chlorogenic.

Medicinal Uses: The plant confers various health benefits, viz treat malaria, psoriasis, allergies, dysentery, urinary tract infection, diarrhoea, rheumatic pain, skin inflammation, asthma, nausea, vomiting, neuralgia and dizziness. This plant is traditionally utilized for the treatment of migraine headaches, toothaches, insect bites, infertility, rheumatoid arthritis, stomachaches, fever, and problems with menstruation and labor during childbirth. It exhibits anti-cancer activity, cytotoxicity activity, antioxidant activity, anti-inflammatory activity, antimicrobial activity, wound healing activity, pesticidal activity, hypoglycemic activity and thrombolytic activity. The plant is used as antifeedant, antifungal, antimalarial, insecticidal and antiviral agent. Ethnobotanically, it is used to treat inflammation, skin rashes, herpes, eczema, rheumatic pain, cold, heart trouble and gynaecological disorders. Flower extract is used in antitumour activity.

Poisonous Parts: Leaves and seeds.

Toxic Constituents: Parthenin, hymenin, anbrosin, hysterin.

Poisonous Symptoms: Whole plant is poisonous. Leaves, flowers, fruits and seeds cause allergic dermatitis and eczema on contact. The plant when eaten by animals causes diarrhoea followed by death with acute ulceration in the liver, gastrointestinal tracts and kidney. It poses danger to the farm animals particularly in drought condition. When human beings frequently come in contact with this plant it may cause allergy, eczema, black spots, respiratory malfunction, blisters around eyes, burning rings, blisters over skin, redness of skin and asthma and dermatitis in cattle and domestic animals due to the presence of toxin parthenin. The presence of *Parthenium hystrophorus* pollen grain inhibits fruit set in brinjal, tomato, beans, etc and is also capable for bitter milk disorder in livestock fed on grass mixed with its leaves.

Contact with the plant results in severe allergy, rashes, inflammation, peeling of skin in both humans and animals. Humans exposed to this plant for increased period manifest the symptoms of asthma, allergic rhinitis, eczema, black spots, hay fever, skin inflammation, burning and blisters around eyes. The plant also causes diarrhoea, severe popular erythematous eruptions, choking and breathlessness. The plant also causes systemic toxicity in livestock, loss of skin pigmentation, dermatitis, alopecia and diarrhoea. The plant is considered to be a cause of a spectrum of clinical patterns: allergic respiratory problems, contact dermatitis, mutagenicity in human and cattle.

Pedilanthus Tithymaloides (L.) Poit
Family: Euphorbiaceae

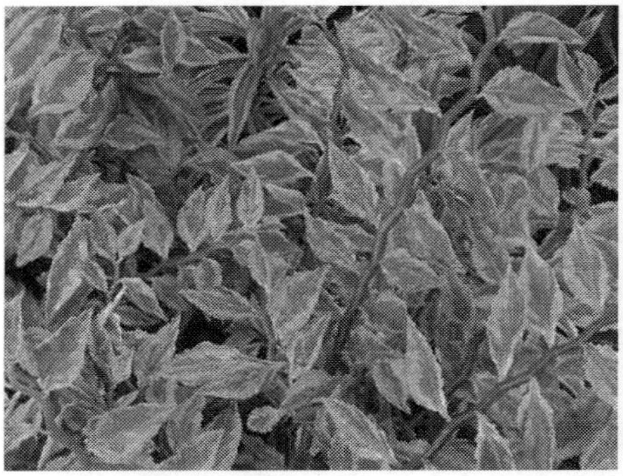

Vernacular Names: *Redbird cactus, Christmas candle, Devil's backbone* (English), *Kannatikalli* (Tamil), *Vilaayathi shera* (Marathi), *Kantapala, Kancipala* (Telugu), *Vilayatikharsani* (Gujarati).

Botanical Description: Succulent shrub with milky juice, 1m height, stems green. The fleshy tubular stems are thin pencil like, grow zig zag and produce thick dark green. Leaves alternate, fleshy, cordate, pointed, simple, green or white edged. Flowers red and clustered at the ends of branches fruit capsule.

Flowering and Fruiting: November - May

Distribution: Tropical America and India.

Propagation: By seeds, stem-tip cuttings and stem cuttings.

Parts Used: Leaves, latex and stem.

Phytochemical Constituents: The plant contains steroids, unsaturated steroids. The leaf of the plant include phenols, terpenes, quercitin, flavonoids, steroids, terpenoids and isoquercitrin, diterpene, pedilstatin, pedilanthain, kaempferol, scopoletin.

Medicinal Uses: The plant is used as antiviral anticancer, antitumoral, abortive agent and is used to treat sore throat. It also exhibits antibacterial, antifungal properties. Latex is used in treating piles, veneral and skin disorders. The plant is used as antiseptic, antioxidant, antimicrobial, anti-inflammatory, antimycobacterial and mosquito larvicidal agent. The leaves are used for wound healing activity, mouth ulcers, asthma, vineral diseases, headache, larvicidal activity. The leaf decoction is used in abdominal disorder. The stem is used as an abortifacient, as antivenom for snake bite and also as remedy for rheumatism. The root is a potent emetic.

Poisonous Parts: Milky sap from entire parts.

Toxic Constituents: Diterpene esters.

Poisonous Symptoms: Latex and root is poisonous and causes vomiting, skin inflammation and skin itching. The latex is injurious to eyes. It causes irritation of the throat and mouth, diarrhea and vomiting when ingested, rash, skin irritation, blistering and eye irritation upon contact.

Plumbago Zeylanica L.

Family: Plumbaginaceae

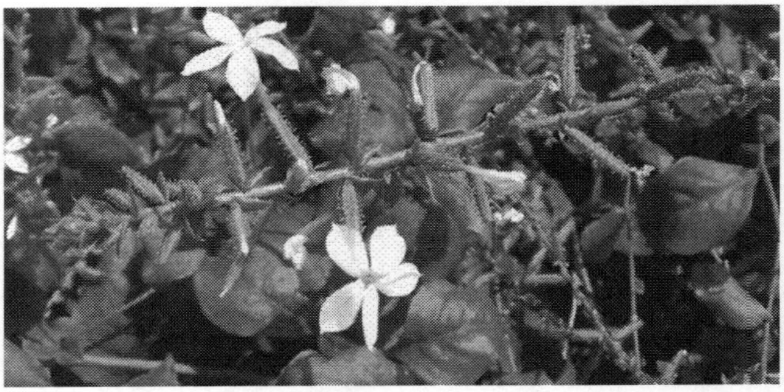

Vernacular Names: *Plumbago, White leadwort, Chitrak* (English), *Chitrak, Lechkuro* (Hindi), *Bogaagechita* (Assamese), *Ogni* (Odisha), *Telhidak angouba* (Manipuri), *Safaid-sitarak* (Bengali), *Chitramulika* (Kannada), *Vellakoduveli, Kodiveli, Tumpakoduveli* (Malayalam), *Chithiramoolam, Kodivaeli, Chita, Chittiri, Chittira* (Tamil), *Chitro* (Gujrati), *Chitramul* (Marathi), *Chitramulamu, Agnimatha* (Telugu), *Agnimata, Agnika* (Sanskrit).

Botanical Description: Much branched, evergreen shrub that reaches upto 2 m height. Dark green leaves are ovate, apex acutely apiculate, petiole to 1.2 cm. Flowers are white in colour terminal, bisexual, rachis glandular, bracteols ovate, acuminate calyx are white with 5 lobes ovate to lanceolate, 1-1.2 cm tubular densely covered with stalked sticky glands. Corolla are tubular, slender, white, 1-1.3 cm long, tubular, densely covered with stalked glands. Stamens 5, unilocular stigma 5 forked, ovary superior, capsule oblong, pale yellow to brown in colour. Seeds are cylindric, flat and dark brown in colour.

Flowering and Fruiting: Throughout the year

Distribution: Native to South East Asia, India, Germany, Africa and Malaysia.

Propagation: By stem cuttings and seeds.

Parts Used: Leaves, root bark, root and seeds.

Phytochemical Constituents: It contains plumbagin. The plant contains a variety of notable chemical compounds. Various parts of the plant possess alkaloids, anthraquinones, cardiac-glycosides, phlobatinnins, naphthaquinones, steroids, triterpenoids, amino acids, tannins, glycosides, saponins, flavonoids, gums, mucilage, phenolic compounds, carbohydrates, coumarins, fixed oil and fats and proteins. Of all the phytoconstituents plumbagin is the principle active compound. The roots contain naphthoquinones, plumbagin, composed naphthoquinones, like plumbagin, 3-biplumbagin, chloroplumbagin, elliptone, chitranone, chittanone, maritinone, droserone. The coumarins sesselin, 5-methoxyseselin, suberosin and xanthyletin. The flowers contain plumbagin, glucose and zeylanone. The leaves contain plumbagin and chitanone. The stem contains plumbagain, zeylanone, isozelanone, sitosterol, campesterol, stigmasterol and dihydroflavinol-plumbaginol.

Medicinal Uses: The plant is used in treatment of dysentery, piles, itching, leucoderma, intestinal troubles, inflammation, disease of the liver upon consumption. The leaves are used in treating scabies, diseases of the spleen, rheumatitis and it acts as an aphrodisiac. Root bark is used as an anti-periodic. The root can act as an abortifacient and vesicant and its acro-narcotic poison can cause abortion. The seed is useful in digestion, and serves as antiseptic, anti-parasitic, caustic and stimulant. The root paste is applied externally to painful rheumatic areas, chronic and itchy skin ailments. It has been used as a medicine for skin ailments, infections and intestinal worms viz. scabies, leprosy, hookworm, acne, ringworm, dermatitis and ulcers. The plant also exhibits antibacterial, antifungal, anti-inflammatory, hepatoprotective, larvicidal, anti-diabetic, anti-cancer, anti-fertility, immunosuppressive, wound healing and antioxidant properties. The whole plant, the roots and powder of the roots are used in treating malaria, fever, dyspepsia, diarrhoea, piles and skin disorder.

Poisonous Parts: Root

Toxic Constituents: Plumbagin

Poisonous Symptoms: Intake of root decoction causes severe skin inflammation, skin itching and gastrointestinal poison. The root of *Plumbago zeylamica* has been reported to be a powerful poison when given internally or applied to ostium uteri, causes abortion. Plumbagin may serve as a potential compound in synthetic insecticides.

Plumeria Rubra L.

Family: Apocynaceae

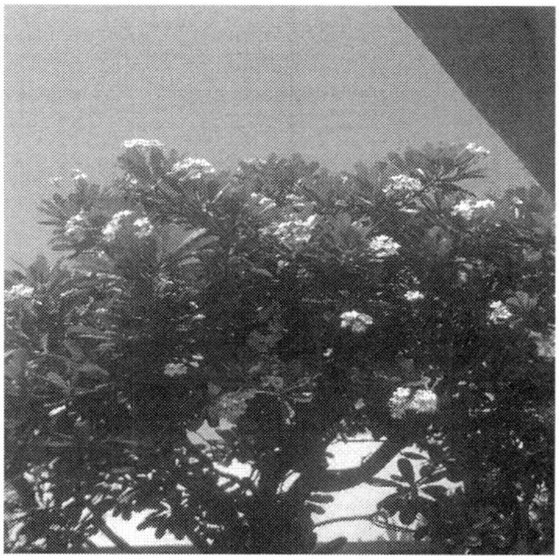

Vernacular Names: *Temple tree, Frangipani plant, True frangipani* (English), *Lal champa, Golainchi* (Hindi), *Segappu arali* (Tamil), *Dalan phul* (Bengali), *Kshirachampa* (Sanskrit), *Nuruvavahaalu* (Telugu), *Devaganigile* (Kannada), *Ezha-champakam* (Malayalam), *Rhada champo* (Gujarati).

Botanical Description: A spreading shrub or small tree. It grows up to 9 m height with 12 m spread. Leaves are alternate, simple petiole undissected, ovate shape or elliptic. It has a dense succulent trunk and sausage – like blunt branches, red or pink colour, spreading cymes fruits elongated. The flowers are terminal, 20-60 winged seeds are present.

Flowering and Fruiting: August - December

Distribution: Central America, India, Mexico, Colombia, Venezuela, Pakistan and Bangladesh.

Propagation: By seeds and stem cuttings

Parts Used: Leaves, roots, bark, fruit and flower

Phytochemical Constituents: The stem bark contains fulvoplumierin and plumierides. The leaves contain alkaloid, steroid, gum, sugar and tannins. The flowers contain volatile components including 1,1 diethoxyethane, 6-methyl 5 heptan-2-01, benzaldehyde, methyl benzolate, tricycle octane, linalool, gerniol, citral, naphthalene, nerolidol, methyl 3-propenylbenzoate, methyl salicylate and benzyl benzoate. The pod contains flavonoids, tannins, steroids, alkaloids, saponins and anthraquinone.

Medicinal Uses: In traditional medicinal method, various parts of this plant are used in treating large variety of ailments, leprosy, asthma, fever, diabetes, ulcers, rheumatism, inflammation, constipation. It possesses anticancer, antioxidant, anthelmintic, antimicrobial, anti-inflammatory properties. The leaves are used in treating bronchitis, cold, cholera, cough, ulcers, leprosy, rheumatism, inflammations, and serve as antifungal, antimicrobial, antipyretic and stimulant. Roots and bark are traditionally utilized to promote menstruation, asthma, ease constipation and reduce fever, leprosy. It is laxative, carminative and thermogenic. Fruit is used to treat abortifacient. The flowers are used in curing dysentery, haemophilia, cough, acute enteritis and constipation.

Poisonous Parts: Plant parts with milky latex

Toxic Constituents: Alkaloids, steroids and tannins

Poisonous Symptoms: Milky latex is poisonous, causes irritation of the skin, pink rash and dermatitis.

Punica Granatum L.

Family: Puniceae / Lythraceae

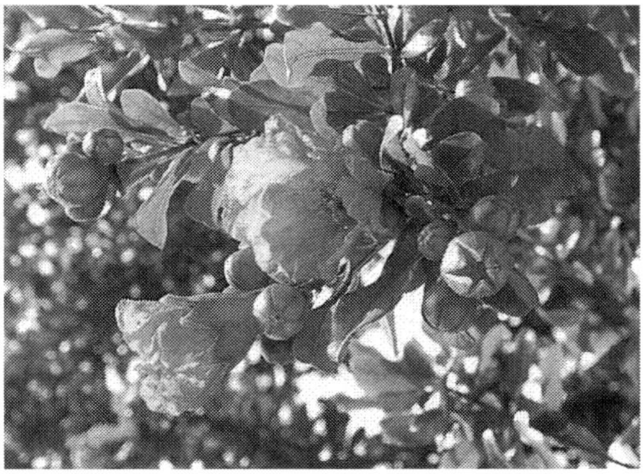

Vernacular Names: *Pomegranate* (English), *Dadima* (Sanskrit), *Madulai* (Tamil), *Danimma* (Telugu), *Dalimba* (Kannada), *Matalam* (Malayalam), *Dalim* (Bengali), *Anar* (Hindi), *Dadam* (Gujarati), *Daalimb* (Marathi)

Botanical Description: A large deciduous shrub or small tree, normally with multiple stems, grows 5-8 m tall. The deciduous leaves are shiny and about 8.1 cm long, flowers orange-red trumpet-shaped, ruffled petals. The flowers are about 5.6 cm long. The fruit is globose, 5.4-7.9 cm in diameter and shiny reddish or yellowish green when mature, fruit berry, numerous seeds.

Flowering and Fruiting: Throughout the year

Distribution: India, Russia, China, Japan, Morocco, Spain, Turkey, Tunisia, Cyprus, Egypt, Pakistan, Bangladesh, USA and Africa

Propagation: By seeds and stem cuttings

Parts Used: Seeds, leaves, immature fruit, fruit rind and flowers

Phytochemical Constituents: The plant contains ellagic acid, Punicic acid, ellagitannins, flavonoids, flavones, anthocyanins, anthocyanidins and estrogenic flavonols, tannins punicalagin, cyanidin, delphinidin, hydroquinone pyridinium and pelargonidin. Saponins, steroids, carbohydrate, alkaloids, protein and amino acids. Many fatty acids, triterpenes, sterols and phenolic compounds, palmitic acid, ethyl palmitate and ethyl oleate. The seed oil contains punicic acid, ellagic acids, other fatty acids, sterols. Pericarp contains phenolic punicalagins, gallic acid and other fatty acids, catechin, flavones, anthocyanidins, flavonones. The leaves contain tannins, flavones, glycosides, including apgenin and luteolin. The flowers contain ursolic acid, triterpenoids, gallic acid, including asistic acid and maslinic acid. Bark and roots contain several piperidine alkaloids, punicalagin, punicalin and ellagitannins.

Medicinal Uses: Seed decoction is used to treat syphilis. Fruit juice is used to cure diarrhoes and jaundice. The juice of the flowers is utilized to manage nose bleeds. Flowers are used to treat diarrhea, heal ulcers, cut wound, bronchitis, diabetes, digestive problems. It is used as astringent, men sex power reconstituent, hemostatic, antiviral, antifungal, antibacterial, anticancer, anti-inflammatory agent and as tonic. It exhibits antidiabetic, antioxidant and hepatoprotective properties. Decoction of the flower is utilized in cases of oral and throat inflammations. The ripe fruit is diuretic, tonic, astringent, laxative, used in brain diseases and chest troubles. It is useful in the cure of leprosy, dyspepsia, snake bite. The fresh fruit is used as refrigerant and can lower fever; leaves, seeds, roots and bark possess antispasmodic, hypotensive and anthelmintic properties.

Poisonous Parts: Bark and leaves

Toxic Constituents: Alkaloid and pelletierine

Poisonous Symptoms: Intake of leaves by human causes vomiting, diarrhea, nausea, headache, dimness of vision, dizziness and greatest muscular weakness followed by paralysis. Cerebral symptoms such as drowsiness, Vertigo and coma may supervene. Intake of immature leaves by livestock causes diarrhoea, vomiting, ulcers of mouth and throat, extreme fever, death within two or four days.

Rauvolfia Serpentina (L.) Benth. ex. Kurz.
Family : Apocynaceae

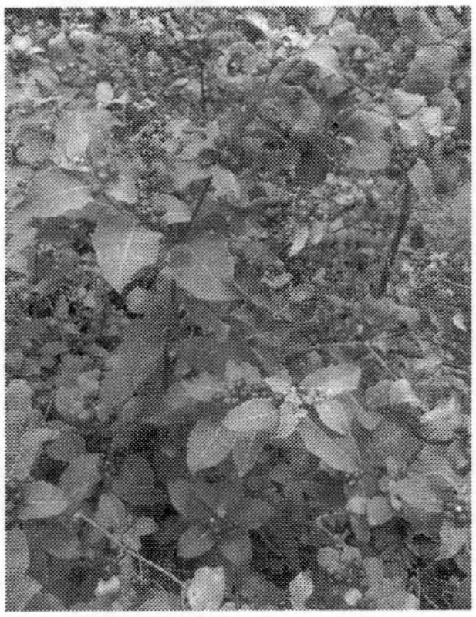

Vernacular Names: *Rauvolfia snake root, Indian snake root, Serpentine root (English), Sarpagandha* (Sanskrit), *Chota chand, Chandrabhaga* (Hindi), *Sarpagantha, Sutranbhi* (Kannada), *Patalagandhi, Sarpaganthi* (Telugu), *Sarpagandhi, Amalpori* (Malayalam), *Chivanamelpodi, Sarpaganthi* (Tamil), *Karki, Chandra* (Marathi), *Chandra* (Bengali), *Aracchoritia* (Assamese), *Dhan-barua* (Odia), *Amelpodee* (Gujarati), *Bhungmaraja* (Arunachal Pradesh).

Botanical Description: An erect, evergreen, perennial, glabrous, undershrubs, 0.6-2m height, bark white, roots tuberous, pale brown, rootstock woody and thick, bark ashy white, thin, latex water, branchlets hairless. Leaves 3-4 in a whorl or sometimes opposite, elliptical, obvate or lanceolate, acuminate, 8-14 x3.6 cm base gradually tapering, apex acuminate, margin entire, papery, hairless, with distinct stalk; lateral nerves 8-14 pairs, cymes long, peduncle rounded rarely recemose. Several flowered, flowers bisexual, in terminal or axillary umbellate cymes. White with pale purple shade about 2.1 x 1.2 cm, flowers white or pinkish, calyx small, corolla tube often curved, throat hairy, fruiting shortly, drupes 0.70 cm broadly oblique ovoid; drupes black, united in their lower half, stalkless, fleshy, ovoid, about 7.1 mm long, hairless, shiny, purplish black when ripe, seed 1, ovoid.

Flowering and Fruiting: March - December

Distribution: India, Nepal, Burma, Thailand, Indonesia, Sri Lanka, Philippines, Cambodia and Bangladesh

Cultivation: By seeds, stem cuttings and root cuttings

Parts Used: Roots and leaves

Phytochemical Constituents: The root, stem and leaves contain a number of alkaloids of which rescinnamine, deserpidine, reserpine, ajmaline, ajamalicine, α-yohimbine, neoajmalin, serpentine, diserpine, ajmalinine, asmaline, iso-ajmaline, sepentinine, alstonine, yohimbine, rauwolfinine, renoxidine, reserpiline, reserpin, rescin-namine, reserpinine, sarpagine, serpentinine, 3-epi-yohimbine, tetraphyllicine, resin, starch, wax, ophioxylin. *N*b-methylajmaline (1), *N*b-methylisoajmaline (2), 3-hydroxysarpagine (3), rohimbinic acid (4), isorauhimbinic acid (5), a new iridoidglucoside, 7-epiloganin (6), and a new sucrose derivative, 6′-0-(3,4,5-trimethoxy benzoyl) glomeratose A (7). Reserpine is an indole alkaloid. Chemically it is (3β, 16β, 17α, 18β, 20α) -11, 17-dimethoxy-18 [(3,4,5-trimethoxy-benzoyl)-oxyl] yohimban - 16-carboxylic acid methyl ester or 3,4,5-trimethoxybenzoyl methyl reserpate. Rauvoxine, rauvoxinine, vomalidine, sandwichine, rauwolfinine, purpeline, seredamine, deserpidene, aricine, neosarpagine, mitoridine, picrinine, obscuridine, rauwolfine, raunamine, raucaffridine, samatine, β-yohimbine, isoraunescine, alkaloid A, alkaloid D, alkaloid PR1, alkaloid PR2, alkaloid PR3 and chandrine. The leaves also contain flavonoids, phenols, tannins and alkaloids.

Medicinal Uses: The plant is used in treating mental disorders, snake bite, insect sting and is used as sedative. Root is useful for the treatment of epilepsy, asthma, acute stomachache, painful delivery, high blood pressure. It is used as an antidote to the bites of poisonous reptile like snakes, dysentery and other painful affections of the intestinal canal. It is used to treat insomnia, cholera, colic, fever, skin disorders. The plant is useful for treating mental sickness, snake bite, insect and animal bite, hypertension, gastrointestinal disorders, schizophrenia, circulatory disorders, malaria, asthma, scabies, eye diseases, pneumonia, body pain, spleen diseases, AIDS, veterinary diseases, headache, body ache, jaundice, blood pressure and as tranquilizer. The plant is also used as sedative, hyphotic and reducing blood pressure. Roots are useful in traditional medication as a valuable cure for various complex disorders e.g. epilepsy, hypochondria, insomnia, high blood pressure, excitement, anxiety, schizophrenia, insanity and other diseases of the central nervous system. The root decoction of this plant is also used to hasten the expulsion of the fetus, diarrhoea, colic, dysentery and cholera, to treat painful affection of bowels.

Poisonous Parts: Roots

Toxic Constituents: Reserpine, reserpidine, reserpinine and serpentine.

Poisonous Symptoms: Consumption of root is poisonous causing stomach upset, vomiting.

Ricinus Communis L.

Family: Euphorbiaceae

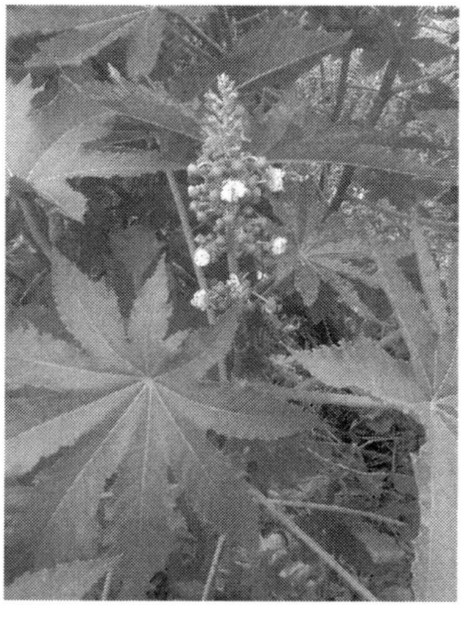

Vernacular Names: *Castor bean, Castor oil plant, Wonder tree* (English), *Erandi, Arandi* (Hindi), *Veranda, Bheranda* (Bengali), *Amanakku, Kottaimuthu* (Tamil), *Chittamankku, Aavanakku* (Malayalam), *Haralu, Oudla* (Kannada), *Amudamuchettu* (Telugu), *Era-gach* (Assamese), *Kege* (Manipuri), *Eranda* (Sanskrit), *Erand* (Marathi).

Botanical Description: Shrub like herb, stems 1 to 12m high, branched, green to reddish or purple, leaves alternate, simple, long stalked, 15 to 45 cm wide and palmately lobed with 6 to 12 long lobes which are toothed on the margins, green or reddish. It has clusters of seed pods, green or red and covered with fleshy spines. The seeds contained in the pods are 3 per capsule, about 1.7 to 2.8 cm across, elliptical glossy, black or white or usually mottled with grey, black brown and white. The seeds have a pleasant taste. The flowers are borne in terminal panicle like inflorescences of green.

Flowering and Fruiting: Throughout the year

Distribution: Native from Tropical Africa, Thailand, Brazil, India, USA, Rumania, Ethiopia, USSR, South Africa, Tanzania and Paraguay. It is now growing in tropical, subtropical and temperate areas.

Propagation: By seeds and vegetative mode

Parts Used: Seeds

Phytochemical Constituents: Ricins, beta carotene, ellagic acid, ricinine, indoleacetic acid, coumarin, lupeol, stigmasterol, quercetin, chlorogenic acid, casebene, tannins, campesterol, brasicasterol, ricinus, agglustinis, seed saponins, kaempferol flycoside, hyperuside epicutechin, glycoproteins, vitamins B1 and B6, beta-amyrin, N-demethylricine, quinic acid, hemaglutinin, 5-dehydro-avenasterol, ricinolein, alkaloids, flavonoids, -3-0-β-D-xylopyranoside, kaempferol-3-0-β-rutinoside and quercetin-3-0-β-rutinoside, flavonol-3-glycosides, xylosides, glucosides and rutinosides of kaempferol and quercetin.

Medicinal Uses: Small quantity of seed oil is used to treat constipation. The seed oil is also used as a purgative. Bark infusion is used to cure rashes and skin inflammations. Intake of the juice with water is taken internally to treat boils and tumours. It exhibits antioxidant activity, antitumour activity, bone regeneration activity, anti-asthmatic, anti-inflammatory activity. It can serve as analgesic, antipyretic and cardiac tonic. Leaf paste is used as poultice on sores, gout or rheumatic swellings. Decoction of root is given in lumbago. All parts of the plant are poisonous, especially the seeds and leaves.

Poisonous Parts: All parts of the plant are poisonous, especially the seeds and leaves

Toxic Constituents: Recine, recinine, phytotoxin as lectin, ricin, simple protein Toxalbumin, crystalline principle ricinine, the poisonous taxalbumin ricin.

Poisonous Symptoms: Intake of high doses of seed oil is fatal with symptoms of colic, vomiting and gastroenteritis. Two to four seeds can confirm high or even fatal, allergic response of serious sensitivity. Other symptoms include burning sensation in throat and mouth, diarrhea, abdominal pain, gastroenteritis, weakness of body and pulse. Digestive tract shows hemorrhages, liver and kidney damage. Larger quantities of seed oil is poisonous causes diarrhea, weakness of body and slow irregular pulse, kidney and liver damage, abdominal pain, allergic reaction of large sensitivity and vomiting in small amount, death. The young leaves when eaten by goats causes severe diarrhea followed by death. The beans are poisonous to horses, fowls, pigs, sheep and man.

Solanum Nigrum L.

Family: Solanaceae

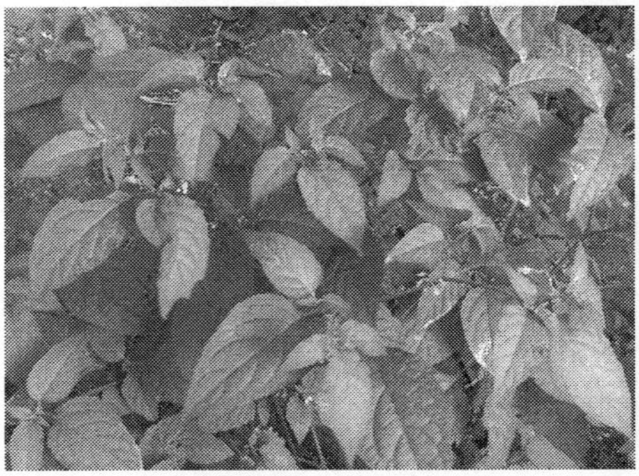

Vernacular Names: *Black-berry night shade, Night shade, Poison berry, Black nightshade* (English), *Makoy, Kabaiya, Gurkkamai, Mokoi* (Hindi), *Kakmaci, Bahutikta, Bhuphala* (Sanskrit), *Milagutakkali, Manattakkali* (Tamil), *Karintakali, Karimthakkali, Manathakkali* (Malayalam), *Kakarundi* (Kannada),

Kamanci, Gajjucettu, Kacci, Kaccipandu (Telugu), *Leipungkhanggu* (Manipuri), *Makoya* (Urdu), *Lghukavali* (Marathi).

Botanical Description: An annual or perennial, unarmed herb up to 1 m tall and with glandular hairs, branched and usually erect. The leaves are alternate, dark green, ovate, nearly entire, deep green with an indented margin and acuminate at the tip. Inflorescences are extra-axillary umbels, the calyx cup-shaped, the corolla is white, 10 lobes ovate-oblong, pubescent abaxially, filaments are 1-1.6 mm long; anthers are 2.6-3.6 mm long. Fruit is many-seeded. The berries are green at early stage and turn to orange or black when ripened. Seeds yellow to dark brown.

Flowering and Fruiting: December – April.

Distribution: Africa, USA, India, Pakistan, Nigeria, Bangladesh, China, Nepal and Sri Lanka

Propagation: By seeds

Parts Used: Whole plant

Phytochemical Constituents: Leaf is a luxuriant principle of nictonic acid, vitamin C and riboflavin. Besides these, B-carotene and citric acid are present. Fruits yield fructose and glucose, vitamin C and B-carotene. The young green fruit of the plant contains four steroidal glyco-alkaloids such as solamargine and α and β - solanigrine and entirely contains solasodine. The plant contains saponin, tannins, alkaloid, protein, flavonoids. Glycoalkaloids, glycoproteins and polysaccharides, polyphenolic compounds such as catechin, gallic acid, protocatechuic acid, caffeic acid, rutin, naringenin and epicatechin are also present.

Medicinal Uses: The plant is used to treat many ailments such as fever, pain, inflammation and enteric disorders. It is a diuretic, antioxidant, anti-inflammatory, anti-ulcer, anticancer, antibacterial, antifungal, cytotoxic, antiulcerogenic, hepatoprotective and antipyretic agent, anti-convulsant. It is also used to manage sexually transmitted ailments. All parts of this plant are utilized in the traditional medication as a cure for treating several diseases like asthma, cold, cough, mycotic infection, skin diseases and liver problem. It is useful for treating vomiting, leprosy, nasal catarrh, dyspepsia, rheumatism. It is used as anodyne, laxative cardiotonic, depurative, febrifuge, tonic and expectorant. The leaves are useful in stomach complaints, fever and dysentery. The juice of the leaf is useful in ulcers and various kinds of skin disorders.

Poisonous Parts: Whole plant, especially fruit and immature berries

Toxic Constituents: Solanine alkaloid and steroids, glycoalkaloids, solamargine, solasonine and solamine

Poisonous Symptoms: The plant contains the poisonous solanine. It is mainly present in the berries, but also present in the stem and leaf. The plant is toxic to cattle, sheep, goats causing severe vomiting and death. Intake of the unripe green berries causes vomiting, abdominal pain, loss of appetite, blood stained feces, diarrhea, sweating, fever, drowsiness and confusion. Death from ingesting plant parts results from respiratory failure and arrhythmias.

Solanum Virginianum L.

Family: Solanaceae

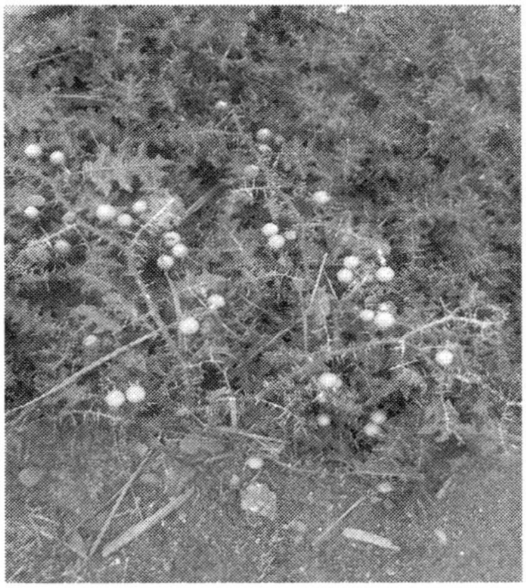

Vernacular Names: *Yellow berried nightshade, Wild egg plant, night shade plant* (English), *Katai* (Hindi), *Kandankattiri* (Tamil), *Kantkari* (Bengali), *Dorall ringani* (Marathi), *Bhoyasingani* (Gujarati), *Ankranti, Bheji begum* (Odisha), *Nella molunga, Pinnamulaka, Callamulaga* (Telugu), *Kantakari* (Assamese), *Kandankattiri* (Malayalam), *Nelagulla* (Kannada), *Kandyall, Warumba, Chhoti mauhari* (Punjabi), *Leipungkhanga* (Manipuri), *Dhavani, Ksudra, Kantokari, Nidigdha, Kantakarika, Dusparsa, Agnidamani* (Sanskrit).

Botanical Description: A prickly diffuse bright green perennial herb woody at the base, 1.5-3 m height. The stem is greenish grey with innumerable spines. Leaves elliptic or ovate, sinuate or subpinnatified, obtuse or subacute, stellately hairy on both sides, armed on the midrib and often on the nerves with lengthy yellow sharp prickles. Flowers are in cymes, bright blue, calyx tube is short, globose and lobes linear-lanceslate, densely hairy and prickly corolla purple, lobes deltoid, acute and hairy outside. Anther filament is lengthy, glabrous and anthers open by a pore. Ovary is ovoid. The fruits are glabrous, globular berries, green and white strips when young but becomes yellow when matured, green-blothed and surrounded by enlarged calyx. Seeds are glabrous, several.

Flowering and Fruiting: May - August

Distribution: South East Asia, Malaysia, Tropical Australia, India, Pakistan, Sri Lanka and Bangladesh

Propagation: By seeds

Parts Used: Whole plant

Phytochemical Constituents: Steroidal alkaloid solasodine is the essential alkaloid. Fruit contains solasodine, solarnargine, solasonine, solanocarpine, solanocarpidine and betasolmargine. Dry fruit yielded traces of neochronogenic, chronogenic, caffeic acids and isochlorogenic. The petals contain sitosterol, apigenin and stamens gave quercetin diglycoside. The plant yielded steroidal constituents such as sitosterol, cycloartenol, cycloartanol, glucoside, cholesterol, campesterol, stigmasterol, stigmasterol glucoside, solamargine, beta-solamargine, coumarins, esculin, scopoletin, scopolin and esculetin.

Medicinal Uses: The plant is used in treating throat infections and other inflammatory problems. The fruits are known for many medicinal uses like antipyretic, laxative, anthelmintic, anti-inflammatory, anti-asthmatic and aphrodisiac potentialities. The paste of the fruit is applied externally to the affected area for curing swellings and pimples. Several parts of the plant has high medicinal value. It is used in treating several ailments like fever, heart diseases, cough, asthma, chest pain. It has molluscicidal and insecticidal properties. Fruit juice is utilized in treating rheumatism and sore throats. The decoction of the plant is used in treating gonorrhea. The leaves are applied locally to relieve pain. This perennial herb is used in stopping vomiting, hair fall, leprosy, itching, bronchial asthma, skin diseases, cough, chest pain and scabies. The plant is also useful in treating edema, wounds and cardiac disorders. The plant extract has stomachic, antipyretic, carminative, laxative, febrifuge and aphrodisiac potentialities. Fruits, flowers and stem are bitter and carminative. It is also utilized in treating asthma, cough and pains in chest. The juice of the leaves mixed with black pepper is prescribed in treating rheumatism. The seed is used in treatment of toothache, expectorant in cough and asthma. The plant has been utilized traditionally for treating several sickness. The ripe fruits are burnt and fumes are taken for the curing of toothache problems.

Poisonous Parts: Root

Toxic Constituents: Solasonine, solamargine, steroids and alkaloids

Poisonous Symptoms: Root decoction with sugar is given internally to women for abortion of up to 3 to 5 months old foetus. Large doses are poisonous and cause death of women.

Strychnos Nux-vomica L.

Family: Loganiaceae

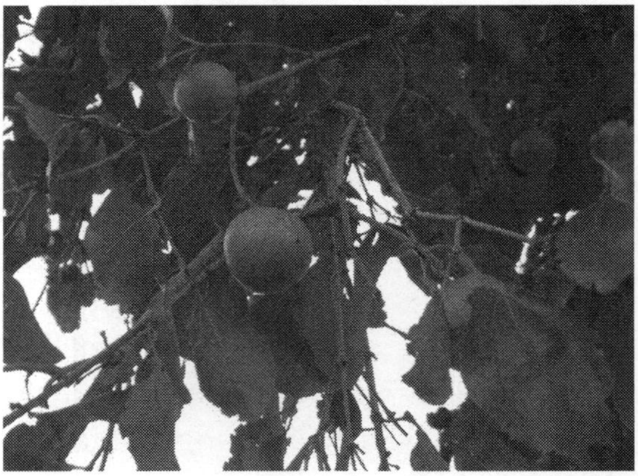

Vernacular Names: *Snake wood, Poison nut, Strychnine plant, Nux-vomica, Crow fig, Poison Nut, Strychnin* (English), *Bailewa, Kajra, Jahar, Kuchla* (Hindi), *Kuchila* (Bengali), *Hemmushti, Ittanji* (Kannada), *Kanjiram, Chamram* (Malayalam), *Kajra, Kuchala* (Marathi), *Kuchla* (Odia), *Chipita, Chutaka, Kapilu* (Sanskrit), *Etti, Kagodi, Kalam,*

Kanjaram, Kancirai (Tamil), *Kuchla muddabir* (Urdu), *Mucidi, Mushti, Mushidi* (Telugu).

Botanical Description: A medium sized tree up to 30 m height, thick trunk, wood is white hard, close grained, root very bitter, branches irregular, covered with a smooth ash-coloured bark, leaves opposite, oval, short stalked, shiny, smooth on both sides. 10 cm long and 7 cm broad, flowers small, greeny-white, funnel shape in small terminal corymbs. Calyx 5-toothed, permanent filaments scarcely any or exceedingly short, inserted over the bottom of the divisions of the corolla, anthers oblong, half within the tube, ovary 2-celled, with many ovules in each cell. Fruit orange colour globose berry, filled with a soft white jelly, seeds 1-4, immerged in the pulp of berry disc-shaped 16 to 32 mm in diameter and 5-7 mm thick, silky hairs.

Flowering and Fruiting: August - January

Distribution: Throughout India, Myanmar, Malaysia, Sri Lanka, China, U.S.A, South East Asia and Africa. It is cultivated in Sudan and Ghana.

Propagation: By seeds.

Parts used: Bark, leaves, seeds and root

Phytochemical Constituents: The whole plant contains strychnine, brucine and alkaloids, strychnicine, glucoside loganin, fatty matter, copper and caffeotanic acid. Seeds contain loganin, N-methyl-Sec-pseudo-β-colubrine, 4-hydroxystrych, P-hydroxybenzoic, vanillic 2-hydroxy-4-methoxy benzoic, sinapic, syringic acids, kaemperol, quercertin and 3'-O-methyquercetin. 12-hydroxy-strychnine, 15-hydroxy-strychnine, α-colubrine, β-colubrine, icajine, 11-methoxy-icajine, novacine, vomicine, pseudostrychnine, pseudobrucine, pseudo-α-colubrine, isostrychnine, igasuric acid, protein and fixed oil.

Medicinal Uses: The plant is used for treating vomiting, insomnia, abdominal pain, constipation, stomach upset, heart diseases, intestinal irritation, depression, eye ailments, circulatory problems, nervous disorders, menopause problems, respiratory illness, digestive problems, inflammations and blood pressure. It is used as aphrodisiac, laxative, diuretic, healing tonic and appetite stimulant. The powdered seeds are remedy for dyspepsia, ulcers, dysentry and fever. The leaves are applied as poultice in the cure of wounds and ulcers. They are useful in treating jaundice, urinary discharges, piles, anaemia, itching, leucoderma, emenagogue, ringworm, paralysis, cures pains in joints and heating appetizer. The root bark is better and is used in treating cholera.

Poisonous Parts: All parts especially seeds.

Toxic Constituents: Strychnine, vomicine and brucine.

Poisonous Symptoms: Intake of leaves, stem bark, fruits and dried ripe seeds are poisonous causing spinal poison, headache, nausea, kidney failure and vomiting dropsy, slow irregular pulse followed by death. 10-15 seeds can kill human.

Urginea Indica (Roxb.) Kunth
Family: Liliaceae

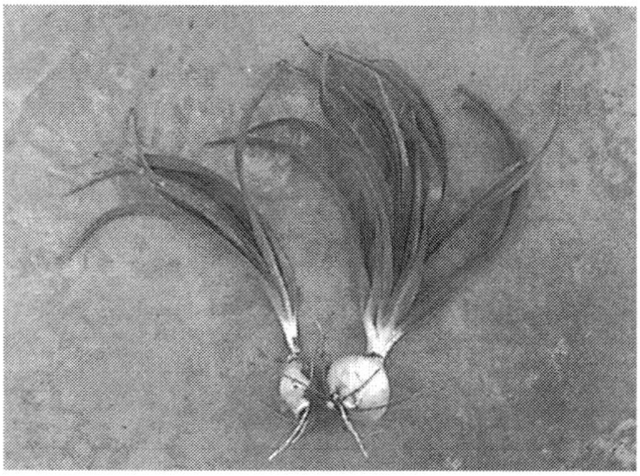

Vernacular Names: *White squill, Indian squill* (English), *Narivengayam* (Tamil), *Junglipiyaz, Ban-Palandu, Ban-Piyazi* (Hindi), *Vanapalandu* (Sanskrit), *nakkavulligadda* (Telugu), *Kattulli* (Malayalam), *Adairirulli* (Kannada).

Botanical Description: A small glabrous, bulbous perennial herb, bulbs tunicated, ovoid or sphere shaped, 6-12 cm long. Leaves linear, acute, subbifavious, flowers greenish white or dirty brown or purplish, in terminal racemes borne on erect, long scapes, capsules ellipsoidal or oblong, seeds several. The seeds in the fruit are white.

Flowering and Fruiting: April - May

Distribution: Endemic to India, Africa, Syria, Greece, Italy, France, Portugal, Morocco, Algeria, Bangladesh, Pakistan and throughout the Plains of India especially in Sandy Soil.

Propagation: By seeds and bulblets.

Parts Used: Bulbs

Phytochemical Constituents: The bulb contains proteins, alkaloids, vitamin C, vitamin E, flavonoids, phenols, glycosides, phenolic compounds, saponins and carbohydrates. It contains quercetin, scillaren A, scillaren B, scillarenin, scilliphaeosidin.

Medicinal Uses: The bulb is used as a source of medicine with biocidal applications. It is used as cardiac stimulant, anticancer agent, expectorant and in curing asthma, dropsy, edema, allergies, gout and rheumatism. The bulb is also useful in treating tumors, cancer, chronic cough, male sterility, psoriasis, swellings, pulmonary troubles, arthritis, incutaneous and subcutaneous parasitic infection. The bulb has various therapeutic significance. It is used in treating chronic bronchitis, leprosy, skin diseases and can serve as diuretic, purgative, digestive, deobstruent, emmenagogue, hypoglycaemic, anthelmintic, cardio-tonic in heart insufficiency, laxative, antioxidant, antiangiogenic, antibacterial and antifungal agent. It is also used to manage headache, disease of nose and scabies.

Poisonous Parts: Bulb

Toxic Constituents: Glycosides, saponins, alkaloids and carbohydrates

Poisonous Symptoms: Greatest consumption of bulb is poisonous and causes blood urine, nausea and strangury. It leads to suppression of urine, gastroenteritis, convulsion of heart and paralysis followed by death.

GLOSSARY OF BOTANICAL TERMS

Achene Minute dry indehiscent fruit containing a particular seed.

Actinomorphic Radially symmetrical, that is capable of section by straight boundaries into three or more similar divisions.

Acuminate With a elongated, tapering point set off rather shortly from the main body.

Acute With a pointed end forming an acute angle, that is less than a right angle.

Adnate United to a member of another order.

Alternate With a single structure of each kind occurring at each level of the axis. E.g. stem. These structures (e.g. branches and leaves) appear alternate on opposite sides of the axis, but actually are spiral in arrangement.

Androphore A stalk or other supporting arrangement under stamens raised above their regular position in the flower.

Angiosperms They are flowering plants with seeds enclosed inside fruits.

Annual A plant completing its life cycle in a year or less.

Anther They are pollen bearing portion of stamen in flower.

Apiculate Terminated by an abrupt, small, flexible point.

Aril A large appendage of the funiculus at the hilum (attachement area) of a seed. It tends to envelop the seed.

Axillary In the axil

Axillary flower A flower in the axil of a bract or a leaf.

Bark They are all the tissues outside the cambium.

Basal leaves Leaves at the lower portion of an herbaceous plant, arising from many nodes separated by exceedingly small internodes occurring at about surface level.

Bearded With long or stiff hairs.

Berry A pulpy or fleshy fruit with more than one seed and formed from either a superior or an inferior ovary. The seeds are embedded in pulpy tissue.

Bifid Divided into 2 parts, bifurcated.

Bilabiate 2-lipped, A bilabiate corolla has petals in two sets, commonly with two in upper and three in the lower.

Bipinnate Pinnate and the first leaflets again pinnate.

Bisexual With two sexes in the same inflorescence or flower.

Bract A modified leaf having flower or an inflorescence in its axis.

Bracteate With bracts

Bracteolate With bractlets

Bracteole Diminutive of bract, a mere scale.

Bracteole Leaf like appendage on the stalk of a flower.

Bractole Diminutive of bract, a mere scale.

Calyx A cup, outer envelope of a flower of the dicotyledons, often scarious or green.

Campanulate Bell-shaped, that is the produce of an inverted church bell.

Capitulum A short head.

Capsule A dry, several-seeded fruit made up of more than one carpel and splitting open lengthwise at maturity.

Carinate With a keel.

Cauline Belonging to the stem or axis.

Climbing Supported by clinging.

Compressed Flattened, particularly side to side.

Corolla The petals of a flower, that is, the inner series (or many series) of the perianth. Each petal has usually a single vascular trace.

Corymb A flat-topped inflorescence.

Corymbose Arranged in corymbs.

Creeping The stem growing along the surface and producing adventitious roots.

Crenate With rounded teeth projecting at right angles to the edge of the leaf.

Crustaceous Hard and brittle in texture.

Culm The false stem of a grass.

Cyme A broad divaricate inflorescence.

Deciduous Trees showing leaf fall in winter season.

Decompound More than once compound.

Decussate In reverse pairs with the rotate pairs projecting at right angles to each other.

Dentate With angular teeth projecting at right angles to the edge of the arrangement.

Didynamous In two pairs, the pairs not being of the same reach.

Digitate Resembling the fingers of a human hand, that is, with various alike structures arising at a general point.

Dioecious Male and female flowers on various plants.

Divaricate Spreading widely, that is divergent.

Drupe A fruit with a fleshy exocarp and a hard, stony endocorp around each seed.

Elliptical In the form of an ellipse, that is, about one and one half times as long as broad, widest at the middle and rounded at both ends.

Endemic Restricted in occurrence to a particular geographical area.

Endocarp The innermost layer of the pericarp.

Entire Without division or toothing of any kind.

Erect Standing upright.

Fascicle A cluster or bundle.

Female Pistil bearing.

Filiform Threadlike, that is elongated, slender and cylindroidal.

Fleshy fruit A fruit with flexible, juicy tissues.

Flora List of plants growing in a particular region.

Florets Individual flowers, very small flowers that make up a very crowded form of inflorescence.

Floriferous Bearing flowers.

Flower The reproductive stem of the angiosperms. Typically it is made up of a calyx of sepals, a corolla of petals, an andrecium of stamens and a gynecium of carpels.

Follicle A dry fruit formed from one carpel, containing more than single seed, and splitting open along the suture.

Fruit The ovary and its contents after the fertilization of the ovules.

Furrowed With longitudinal grooves.

Genus A group of related species or sometimes an individual species.

Glabrescent Initially hairy but later becoming glabrous.

Glabrous Not hairy

Glandular Bearing glands, short cellular organs secreting resins, oils, tars etc.

Globose Spheroidal.

Graft A small piece of meristematic tissue, e.g., a bud or growing shoot, called the scion, is made to unite with a larger established plant, called the stock.

Gynophore A peculiar stalk under a pistil.

Hairy Clothed with hairs.

Hartwood Central mass of xylem become hard as a result of tylosis and no longer support water conduction and help in mechanical support only.

Herb A plant not woody, at least one which is not woody above ground level.

Herbaceous Not woody

Hispid With stiff bristles.

Imparipinnate With a terminal leaflet.

In Vitro In culture

In Vivo Within the organisms

Indehiscent Not opening by pores or valves.

Inflorescence It is a flower cluster.

Involucre One or more whorls of minute leaves.

Irregular Zygomorphic, unsymmetrical

Labiate It refers to a corolla with one or more petals formed into a lip.

Lanceolate Lance-shaped; four to six times as long as broad, broadest toward the basal end, sharply angled at both end and especially the apical end, the sides being curved at least along the broad part.

Latex A milky fluid containing sugars, proteins, alkaloids, oil etc. produced in latex vessels of various plants.

Leaflet A leaf like segment of a compound leaf.

Linear Long and narrow, the sides being parallel and the length at least eight times the width, tending to be an elongated rectangle.

Lineolate Marked with thin lines.

Loculicidal Dehiscent along the midrib of a carpel of an ovary containing more than one chamber and carpel.

Male flower Androceium bearing flower.

Merous In composition, referring to the numbers of parts; as flowers five-merous.

Micropyle A little opening in the integument which forms the outer layer of an ovule or a seed. The pollen tube enters the ovule through this opening.

Midrib The chief rib of a leaf.

Monadelphous In one brotherhood; referring to stamens with their filaments coalescent into a single tube.

Monoecious Female and male flowers on the same plant.

Mucilaginous Slimy, as if covered with mucilage.

Node A joint of the stem, that is, the region which bears a leaf or a pair of or various leaves usually each with a branch or buds in its axil.

Nut A hard, relatively great, indehiscent, 1-seeded fruit.

Nutlet Diminutive of nut.

Oblong Rectangular and longer than wide, the extent roughly two to three times the breadth.

Obovate Ovate but with the close part toward the attachment.

Obovoid Ovoid, but with the attachment at the short end.

Obtuse Abrupt, that is forming an obtuse angle, or somewhat rounded instead of strictly angular

Opposite Inserted at the same level.

Ovary The lower part of the pistil, which contains the ovules or later the seeds.

Ovate Egg-shaped.

Ovule The nucellus containing the embryo-sac and enclosed by 1 or 2 integuments, which after fertilization and subsequent development, becomes a seed.

Panicle A cluster of associated spikes, corymbs or racemes.

Paniculate In a panicle; alike panicle.

Papilionaceous Butterfly like, as corolla of Fabaceae family.

Pappus Calyx modified into hairs.

Pedicel The internode below a flower.

Peduncle The stalk of a cluster of flowers.

Pendulous Hanging downward.

Pentamerous The flowers parts in fives.

Perennial Continuing to grow year after year.

Perianth The floral envelops including both calyx and corolla, no variations into calyx and corolla.

Persistent Remaining attached longer than might be expected.

Petal One member of the arrangement of flower parts forming the corolla.

Petiolate Having a petiole.

Petiole The stalk of a leaf supporting the expanded portion.

Phyllotaxy Arrangement of leaves on stem.

Pistil The organ of a flower which bears ovules and later seeds.

Pod A dry fruit developed from a monocarpellary ovary.

Pollen The spheroidal structures produced in an anther.

Pollinium The waxy body of pollen produced in the milk weed family.

Polysepalous With free sepals.

Prostrate Flat upon the ground.

Pubescent Downy or hairy, usually with fine soft hairs.

Pyriform Pear-shaped.

Raceme It refers to a definite inflorescence, with the main axis bearing stalked flowers which are borne in acropetal succession.

Rachis The axis of a pinnate leaf or of an inflorescence.

Ray A pedicel within an umbel, a ray flower or its corolla.

Ray-flower In the sun flower family or Asteraceae, on of the flowers with a ligulate corolla.

Reniform Bean-shaped, with the attachment in the indentation, the width greater than the extent, the apex rounded.

Reticulate A pattern which arises like a net-work.

Rhizomatous With a rhizome.

Rhizome An elongated underground stem bearing buds in the axils of reduced scale leaves.

Root The lower part of the axis of a angiosperm. It is usually branching and does not bear buds or leaves.

Rootstock An old, incorrect term for rhizome.

Scale A fine, memberanous arrangement; A little more or less triangular leaf; a chaff-like bract; a flattened hair.

Scape Leaflets peduncle arising from the ground; it may bear scales.

Scarious Dry, meager, membranous, non-green and translucent.

Seed A stock of a fertilized ovule, consisting of an integument, an enclosed nucellus, the remains of the megagametophyte, the endosperm and the embryo.

Segment One of the parts of a leaf, calyx, corolla or perianth.

Sepal One of the flower parts of the outer orders, the sepal forming a calyx.

Sessile Without a stalk.

Silky Covered densely with a pressed, soft, straight hairs.

Smooth Not rough, some writers have employed this term incorrectly to mean glabrous.

Solitary Alone.

Species A group of related varieties or often a single unit.

Spike An inflourescence in which main axis is elongated and flowers are sessile.

Spikelet Diminutive of spike; the minute densely bracteate spike of a grass.

Spine A sharp more or less woody or horny outgrowth from a leaf or a part of a leaf, sometimes representing the entire leaf. The term has been applied sometimes to similar outgrowths from the stem.

Stamen The pollen-producing structure of a flowering plant, consisting of an anther and of a filament.

Stem The axis of a plant bearing leaves with buds in their axils. It may be above or below ground.

Stigma The epical portion of a pistil.

Style The narrow part of the pistil bearing the stigma.

Succulent The structure (leaf or stem) much thicker than in most plants; applied as a noun to a plant with succulent parts, especially leaves or stems.

Taxon A category used in classification as for example, a variety, species, genus and family.

Tendril A stem, leaf modified as a branched or unbranched filamentous structure, used by many climbers for attachment to a support by twining or by adhesive terminal disks.

Terete Slender and more or less cylindroidal, approximately circular in cross division, but of varying diameter.

Terminal At the end point.

Testa The seed coat, that is, the hardened mature integument.

Tetramerous With four members, the flower parts in four.

Thorn A pointed shoot, sometimes this term is used interchangeably with spine.

Tomentose Woolly, that is closely covered with matted hairs.

Toothed With smaller projections and indentations alternating along the margin.

Tree A woody plant with a main trunk. Trees in common are greater than shrubs.

Trichome A bristle or hair.

Tripinnate Three times pinnate, that is, with first, secondary and tertiary leaflets.

Triquetrous 3-angled in cross division.

Triquetrous Having three fine or projecting angles.

Truncate Appearing as if cut off at the close.

Tuberculate With tubercles, that is processes.

Tuberous Tuber like in manner or nature.

Tubular Forming an elongate hole cylinder.

Tunic A loose membranous outer skin not the epidermis; the loose membrane about a bulb.

Turbinate Top-shaped, that is, more or less in an inverted cone.

Twiner A climber, which climbs by spirally coiling stems.

Umbel A raceme in which the axis has not elongated, so that the flowers stalks arise at the same point. Thus the flowers are in a head, with the oldest at the outside.

Umbellate Umbelled; pertaining to umbers.

Unilocular 1 chambered ovary.

Unisexual Of only one sex. Descriptive of a flower having only pistils or only stamens, not both.

Valvate Margins of calyx or corolla not overlapping.

Variety The smallet taxon usually recognized.

Whorl A cycle or a verticil, that is, a group of leaves or other structures at a particular.

Zygomorphic (Irregular) Bilaterally symmetrical, often this is described as 'abnormal', especially with reference to corollas.

REFERENCES

1. Abhijit Dey and De, J.N. 20 10. *Rauvolfia serpentina* (L.) Benth. ex. Kurz. – A review. *Asian Journal of Plant Sciences.* 9(6):285-298.

2. Abhijit Dey and De, J.N.2011. Ethnobotanical aspects of *Rauvolfia serpentina* (L.) Benth. ex. Kurz. in India, Nepal and Bangladesh. *J.Med.Plant.Res.* 5(2):144-150.

3. Adediwura, A., Fred-Jaiyesimi and Kola K., Ajibesin. 2014. Ethnobotanical survey of toxic plants and plant parts in Ogun State, Nigeria. *International Journal of Green Pharmacy.* 6:174-179.

4. Adeniran, A.A. and Sonibare, M.A. 2013. *In Vitro* potential anthelmintic activity of bulbils of *Dioscorea bulbifera* L. on earthworms and liverflukes. *J. Pharmacognosy Phytother.* 5(2):196-203.

5. Agbarfor, K.N., Akubugwo, E.I., Ogbashi, M.E., Ajah, P.M. and Ukwandu, C.C. 2011. Chemical and antimicrobial properties of leaf extracts of *Zapoteca portoricensis*. *Res. J.Med. Plant,* 5: 605-612.

6. Agra, M.F., Baracho, G.S., Nurit, K., Bajilio, I.J.L.D. and Coelho, V.P.M. 2007. Medicinal and poisonous diversity of the flora of Cariri paraibano, Brazil. *Journal of Ethnopharmacology.* 111:383-395.

7. Ahmad, N., Fazal, H., Ayaz, M., Abbasi, B.H., Mohammad, I. and Fazal, L. 2011. Dengue fever treatment with *Carica papaya* leaves extracts. *Asian Pacific Journal of Tropical Biomedicine.* 1(4):330-333.

8. Ahmed, S.A., Nazim, S., Siraj, S., Siddik, P.M. and Wahid, C.A. 2011. *Euphorbia neriifolia* Linn: A phytopharmacological review. *International Research Journal of Pharmacy.* 2(5):41-48.

9. Ahmedullah, M. and Nayar, M.P. 1986. Endemic Plants of the Indian Region. Vol.I. Botanical Survey of India, Calcutta.

10. Alagesaboopathi, C. 2009. Ethnomedicinal plants and their utilization by villagers in Kumaragiri Hills of Salem district of Tamilnadu, India. *Afr.J.Traditional Complementary and Alternative Medicines.* 6, 222-227.

11. Alagesaboopathi, C. 2011. Antimicrobial potential and phytochemical screening of *Andrographis affinis* Nees. An endemic medicinal plant from India. *Int. J. Pharm. Sci.* 3:157-159.

12. Alagesaboopathi, C. 2011. Antimicrobial screening of selected medicinal plants in Tamilnadu, India. *African Journal of Microbiology Research,* 5: 617-621.

13. Alagesaboopathi, C. 2012. Poisonous plants of the Salem district of Tamilnadu, Southern India. *Journal of Pharmacy Research.* 5(10):5039-5042.

14. Alagesaboopathi, C. 2013. Endemic Medicinal Plants. MJP Publishers, Chennai.

15. Alagesaboopathi, C. 2014. Medicinal plants used by tribal and non-tribal people of Dharmapuri district, Tamilnadu, India. *Int.J.Curr.Res.Biosci.Plant Biol.* 1(2):64-73.

16. Al-Yahya, M.A. 2000. Preliminary toxicity study on the individual and combined effects of *Citrullus colocynthis* and *Nerium oleander* in rats. *Fitoterapia.* 71:385-391.

17. Anilkumar. 2014. *Parthenium hystrophorus* L. And its impact on living world. *Indian J. Sci. Res.* 4(1):8-14.

18. Apollo, M, Dash S.K. and Padhy S. 2006. Eco-consciousness for poisonous and injurious plants among urban dwellers of Bhubaneswar, Orissa. *J.Hum.Ecol.* 19(4):239-248.

19. Aravind, G., Bhownik, D., Duraivel, S. and Harish, G. 2013. Traditional and Medicinal uses of *Carica papaya. Journal of Medicinal Plants Studies.* 1(1):7-15.

20. Arivudainambi, S. and Baskaran, P. 2004. *Cleistanthus collinus* Benth a potential source of pesticidal value. *Annals of Plant Protection* Sci (India). 12(1):202-203.

21. Aruna, K., Devi Raja Rajeswari, Prabu, K., Ramkumar, M., Chidambaram, R. and Raja Sankar, S. 2014. Quantitative phytochemical analysis of *Oxalis corniculata* L. (Oxalidaceae). *World Journal of Pharmacy and Pharmaceutical Sciences.* 3(3):711-716.

22. Arunachalam, K. and Parimelazhagan, T. 2011. Ethnomedicinal observations among *Hooralis* tribes in Kadambur Hills, (Kalkadambur) Erode district, Tamilnadu. *Global J.Pharmacol.* 5(3):117-121.

23. Arya, V., Yadav, S., Kumar, S. and Yadav, J.P. 2010. Antimicrobial activity of *Cassia occidentalis* L. (Leaf) against various human pathogenic microbes. *Life Sciences and Medicine Research.* LSMR-9. 1-11.

24. Ashwani Kumar, Niketa, Sapna Rani and Somiya Sagwal. 2012. An absolute review on *Oxalis corniculata* Linn. *International Journal of Research in Pharmaceutical and Biomedical Sciences.* 3(3):1173-1188.

25. Atal, C.K. and Kapur, M. 1982. Cultivation and utilization of medicinal plants. Council of Scientific and Industrial Research, Jammu Tawi.

26. Atanu, F.O., Ebiloma, U.G. and Ajayi, E.I. 2011. A review of the pharmacological aspects of *Solanum nigrum* Linn. *Biotechnol. Mol. Biol. Rev.* 6(1):1-7.

27. Ayenigbara, G.O. 2012. Medical utility of *Cannabis sativa. Journal of Pharmacy.* 2(3):460-463.

28. Ayyanar, M. 2013. Traditional herbal medicines for primary healthcare among indigneous people in Tamilnadu, India. *J.Homeop.Ayurv.Med.* 2(5):1-7.

29. Badgujar, S.B. and Mahajan, R.T. 2011. Bioprospecting of *Euphorbia nivulia* Buch. *Indian Journal of Pharmaceutical Science and Research.* 1(1):4-9.

30. Balakrishnan, B.R., Sangameswaran, B. and Bhaskar, V.H. 2010. Effect of methanol extract of *Cuscuta reflexa* aerial parts on hep-

atotoxicity induced by antitubercular drugs in rats. *International Journal of Applied Research in Natural Products.* 3(1):18-22.

31. Balandrin, M.F., Kjocke, A.J. and Wurtele, E. 1985. Natural plant chemicals : *Sources of Industrial and Mechanical Materials Science.* 228:1154-1160.

32. Ballantyne, B., Mars, T.C. and Turner, P. 1995. Fundamentals of Toxicology, General and Applied Toxicology, McMillan Press.

33. Banerjee, A.K. and Ira Banerjee. 1986. A survey of the medicinal plants in Shevaroy Hills. *J. Econ. Tax. Bot.* 8(2):271-289.

34. Bhalke, R.D., Mandole, Y.P. and Mali, N.B. 2009. Phytochemical investigation and effect of various extracts of *Argemone mexicana* (Papaveraceae) leaves onclonidine and halopeeridol – induced catalepsy in mice. *Journal of Pharmacy Research.* 2(4):765-767.

35. Bhaskar, L., and Punjani. 2003. Poisonous plants in the forest areas of Vijaynagar Taluka (North Gujarat). *Journal of Economic and Taxonomic Botany.* 27(1):196-204.

36. Bhatia, H., Manhas, R.K., Kumar, K. and Magotra, R. 2014. Traditional knowledge on poisonous plants of Udhampur district of Jammu and Kashmir, India. *Journal of Ethnopharmacology.* 152:207-216.

37. Bhattacharjee, I., Chatterjee, S.K. and Chandra, G. 2010. Isolation and identification of antibacterial components in seed extracts of *Argemone mexicana* L. (Papaveraceae). *Asian Pac J Trop Med.* 3(7):547-551.

38. Bhuvaneshwari, R., and Balasundaram, C. 2006. Traditional Indian herbal extracts used *In vitro* against growth of the pathogenic bacteria *Aeromonas hydrophila, Islamic Journal of Aquaculture.* 58:89-96.

39. Biala, R.G., Tits, M., Walters, J.N. and Angenot, L. 1996. A new HPLC method for the assay of alkaloid in *Strychnos nux-vomica* and *Strychnos ignatti. Fitoterapia.* 67:163-165.

40. Bigoniya, P. and Rana, A.C. 2009. Subacute effect of *Euphorbia neriifolia* Linn. on hematological, biochemical and antioxidant enzyme parameters of rat. *Acad. J. Plant Sci.* 2(4):252-259.

41. Butler, M.S., and Cooper, M.A. 2011. Antibiotics in the clinical pipeline in 2011. *J.Antibiotics,* 64:413-425.

42. Caius, J.F. 2003. The medicinal and poisonous plants of India, Scientific Publishers, Jodhpur.

43. Carpinella, M.C., Defago, M.T., Valladares, G. and Palacios, S.M. 2003. Antifeedant and insecticide properties of a limonoid from *Melia azedarach* (Meliaceae) with potential use for pest management. *J. Agri.Food Chem.* 51:369-374.

44. Charak, D. 1996. The Charak Samhita explained by K.Sastri and G.N.Chaturvedi, 22nd Rev. Edn. Chaukhamba Bharati Academy, Varanasi.

45. Chaudhuri, P.K. and Thakur, R.S. 1994. *Gloriosa superba* : A review. *Curr.Res. Med. Arom.* Plants. 16:51-64.

46. Chauhan, R., Ruby, K.M., Aasthashori and Jaya Dwivedi. 2012. *Solanum nigrum* with dynamic therapeutic role : A Review. *Int. J. Pharm. Sci. Rev. Res.* 15(1):65-71.

47. Chew, A.L., Jessica, J.J.A. and Sasidharan, S. 2012. Antioxidant and antibacterial activity of different parts of *Leucas aspera. Asian Pacific Journal of Tropical Biomedicine.* 2(3):176-180.

48. Cheze, M., Gaillard, Y. and Pepin, G. 2000. Poisoning by plant material: analytical determination of main toxins by high performance liquid chromatography mass spectrometry, Review of human cases. Analytica munich.

49. Chitra, M., Muga, V., Dhanarasu, S., and Al-hazimi, A.M. 2011. Screening of phytochemical and *In Vitro* activity of *Euphorbia hirta* L. *J. Chem. Pharm. Res.* 3(6):110-114.

50. Chitra, M., Senthilkumar, N. and Asraf Ali, M. 2013. Evaluation of hepatoprotective and antioxidant activity of *Euphorbia cyathophora. Int. J. of Res. in Pharmacology and Pharmacotherapeutics.* 2(3):483-490.

51. Chitra, M., Senthilkumar, N. and Asraf Ali, M. 2014. Antimicrobial and wound healing activities of *Euphorbia cyathophora. International Journal of Pharmacology Research.* 4(1):59-61.

52. Chopra, R.C., Badhwar, R.L. and Ghosh, S. 1984. Poisonous plants of India, Indian Council of Agricultural Research. New Delhi, Vol 1&2.

53. Chopra, R.N., Badhwar, R.L. and Ghosh, S. 1949. Poisonous plants of India. Vol. I. Indian Council of Agricultural Research, New Delhi.

54. Chopra, R.N., Badhwar, R.L. and Ghosh, S. 1965. Leguminosae, In:Kurup, C.R.R. (Ed.). Poisonous plants of India Vol-I. Indian Council of Agriculatural Research, New Delhi.

55. Chopra, R.N., Nayar, S.L. and Chopra, I.C. 1992. *Glossary of Indian Medicinal Plants*, 2nd Edition, Council of Scientific and Industrial Research, New Delhi.

56. Chopra, R.N., Nayar, S.L. and Chopra, L.C. 1956. *Glossary of Indian Medicinal Plants.* Council of Scientific and Industrial Research, New Delhi.

57. Chora, R.N., Bhadwar, R.L. and Ghosh, S. 1949. Poisonous plants of India. Vol. I., ICAR, New Delhi.

58. Choubey, V.B. and Khare, P.K. 2011. An inventory of poisonous plants of Sagar district, Madhya Pradesh, (India). *The Indian Forester.* 137(11):1331-1334.

59. Choudhary, M., Kumar, V. and Sing, S. 2014. Phytochemical and Pharmacological activity of Genus *Plumeria:* An updated review. *International Journal of Biomedical and Advance Research.* 5(6):266-271.

60. Cotto, C.M. 1996. *Ethnobotany : Principle and Application,* John Wiley and Sons, New York.

61. Cowan M.M. 1999. Plant products as antimicrobial agents. *Clin. Microbiol. Rev.* 12:564-582.

62. Dash, G.K. and Murthy, P.N. 2011. Evaluation of *Argemone mexicana* Linn. leaves for wound healing activity. *J.Nat.Prod.Plant. Resour.* 1(1):46-56.

63. David, B.C. and Sudarsanam, G. 2011. Ethnomedicinal plant knowledge and practice of people of Javadhu Hills. *Asian Pacific Journal of Tropical Biomedicine.* 1(supplement 1):579-581.

64. De, B and Datta, P.C. 1988. Alkaloids of *Strychnos nux-vomica* flower, *Plant Medica.* 54(4):363.

65. Deka Manalisha and Kalita Jogen Chandra. 2012. Preliminary phytochemical analysis and acute oral toxicity study of *Mucuna pruriens* Linn. in albino mice. *International Research Journal of Pharmacy.* 3(2):181-183.

66. Desale, M.k., Bhamare, P.B., Sawant, P.S., Patil, S.R. and Kamble, S.Y. 2013. Medicinal plants used by the rural people of Taluka Purandhar, district Pune, Maharashtra. *Indian J. Traditional Knowledge.* 12(2):334-338.

67. Dhale, D.A. and Birarj, A.R. 2010. Preliminary screening of antimicrobial and phytochemical studies of *Jatropha Gossypifolia* L. *Rec. Res. Sci. Tech.* 2(7):24-28.

68. Dias and Sabera Sales, E. 2012. Some poisonous plants of Goa. *J. of Econ. and Taxon. Botany.* 36(2):283-291.

69. Dinesh Dabhadkar and Varsha Zade. 2012. Abortifacient activity of *Plumeria rubra* (Linn) Pod extract in female arbino rats. *Indian J. Exp. Biol.* 50:702-707.

70. Dipankar Chandra Roy and Md. Munan Shaik. 2013. Toxicology, Phytochemistry, Bioactive compounds and pharmacology of *Parthenium hysteroporus. Journal of Medicinal Plants Studies.* 1(3):126-141.

71. Dixon, R.A. 2001. Natural products and plant disease resistance. *Nature*. 411:843-847.

72. Duraipandiyan, V., Ayyanar, M. and Ignacimuthu, S. 2006. Antimicrobial activity of some ethnomedicinal plants used by Paliyar tribe from Tamilnadu, India. *BMC complement Altern. Med.* 6:35.

73. Edewor, T.I. and Usman, L.A. 2012. Cytotoxicity and antibacterial activity of the leaf methanolic extract of *Verbena Hastate. J. Med. Plants Res.* 6(1):55-58.

74. Ekundayo, E.O. and Ekekwe, J.N. 2013. Antibacterial activity of leaves extracts of *Jatropha curcas* and *Euphorbia heterophylla. African Journal of Microbiology Research.* 7(44):5097-5100.

75. Fazal, H., Ahmed, N., Ullah, I., Inayat, H., Khan, L. and Abbasi, B.H. 2011. Antibacterial potential in *Parthenium hysterophorus, Stevia rebaudiana* and *Ginkgo biloba. Pak. J. Bot.* 43(2):1307-1313.

76. Francis Xavier, T., Freeda Rose, A. and Dhivyaa, M. 2011. Ethnomedicinal survey of Malayali tribes in Kolli Hills of Eastern Ghats of Tamilnadu, India. *Indian J Traditional Knowledge*. 10(3):559-562.

77. Fransworth, N.O. 1985. The role of medicinal plants in drug development, London, pp.98.

78. Fransworth, N.R. 1994. Ethnopharmacology and drug development. In: Prance, G.T (Ed.), Ethnobotany and the search for New Drugs wiley, Chichester, 185: pp.42-59.

79. Furler, M., Demuth, D., Atthaus, F.R. and Nageli, H. 2000. Computer supported poisonous plant information system for veterinary medicine. *Schweizer Archiv Fur Tierheilkunde.* 142:323-331.

80. Gaillard, Y., Krishnamoorthy A. and Bevalot F. 2004. *Cerbera odollam* : a 'Suicide tree' and cause of death in the State of Kerala, India. *Journal of Ethnopharmacology.* 95:123-126.

81. Gaire, B.P. and Subedi, L. 2013. A review on the pharmacological and toxicological aspects of *Datura stramonium* L. *Journal of Integrative Medicine.* 11(2):73.

82. Gajalakshmi, S., Divya, R., Divya Deepika, V., Mythili, S. and Sathiavelu, A. 2011. Pharmacological activities of *Annona squamosa* : A review. *International Journal of Pharmaceutical Sciences Review and Research.* 10(2):24-29.

83. Galal, M., Bhashir, A.K., Saliah and Adam, S.E.I. 1991. Activity of water extracts of *Albizia anthelmintica* and *A. lebbek* backs against experimental *Hymenolepis diminuta* infections in rats. *Journal of Ethnopharmacology.* 31: 333-337.

84. Gali, K., Ramakrishnan, G., Kothai, R. and Jaykar, B. 2011. *In-vitro* anti-cancer activity of methanolic extract of leaves of *Argemone mexicana.* Linn. *Int. J. PharmTech. Res.* 3(3):1329-1333.

85. Gamble, J.S. 1936. Flora of the Presidency of Madras Vol. I – III Allard & Co. London. (Reprinted – 1956), Botanical Survey of India, Calcutta.

86. Ganesan, S. 2008. Traditional oral care medicinal plants survey of Tamilnadu. *Natural Product Radiance.* 7(2):166-172.

87. Ghosh, S. and Chattopadhyay, D. 2013. Bioactivity guided isolation of anti-inflammatory analgesic, and antipyretic constituents from teh leaves of *Pedilanthus tithymaloides* (L.) *Med. Chem. Res.* 22:4347-4359.

88. Gopi, J., Khatri, P., Singh, N., Gaud, H., and Rakesh Patel. 2011. Phytochemical and pharmacological potential of *Plumeria rubra* Linn. (Apocyanaceae). *Int. J. Ph. Sci.* 3(1):1162-1168.

89. Govaerts, R. 2001. How many species of seed plants are there. *Taxon.* 50:1085-1090.

90. Greval, S.D.S. 1953. Lyon's Medical Jurisprudence for India. 10th Ed. D.L.H.

91. Harisaranraj, R., Suresh, K. and Saravanababu, S. 2009. Evaluation of the chemical composition *Rauvolfia serpentina* and *Ephedra vulgaris. Advances in Biological Research.* 3(5-6):174-178.

92. Harneet Singh and Surendra Kr. Sharma. 2013. Antidiabetic activity of *Jatropha gossypifolia* Linn. root extracts in alloxan induced diabetic mice. *Int. Res. J. Pharm.* 4(5):210-212.

93. Henry, A.N., Kumari, G.R. and Chitra, V. 1987. Flora of Tamilnadu, India, Series 1: Analysis Botanical Survey of India, Southern Circle, Coimbatore.

94. Hill, A.F. 1989. *Economiuc Botany : A Text Book of Useful Plants and Plant Products,* McGraw Hill Book Company, New York.

95. Hoffimann, J.J., Timmerman, N., McLaughlin, R. and Punnapayak. H. 1993. Potential antimicrobial activity of plants from the South Western United States. *International Journal of Pharmacology.* 31:101-105.

96. Hooker, J.D. 1884. The Flora of British India, L. Reeve and Co Kent.

97. Huang, L., Chen, S. and Yang, M. 2012. *Euphorbia hirta* : A review on its ethnopharmacology, phytochemistry and pharmacology. *J. Med. Plants Res.* 6(39):5176-5185.

98. Hussain, I., Khan, N., Riazullah, Shanzeb, Ahmed, S., Khan, F.A. and Ayaz, S. 2011a. Phytochemical, Physiochemical and antifungal activity of *Eclipta alba. Afr. J.Pharm. Pharmacol.* 5(19): 2150-2155.

99. Hussain, I., Rehman, M.U.K., Riazullah, Muhammed, Z., Khan, K., Khan, F.A., Ullah,Z. and Haider, S. 2011b. Phytochemicals screening and antimicrobial activities of selected medicinal plants of Khyberpakhtunkhwa Pakistan *Afr. J. Pharm. Pharmacol.* 5(6):746-750.

100. Hussain, I., Riazullah, Khan, N., Ayaz, S. Ahmed, S., Shanzab, Ahmed, M., Hasan, P.T. and Khan, F.A. 2011c. Phytochemical and inorganic profile of *Calendula officinale* and *Sonachus asper*. *Afr. J. Pharma Pharmacol.* 5(16): 1813-1818.

101. Ilango, K., Maharajan, G. and Narasimhan, S. 2012. Preliminary phytochemical screening and antibacterial activity of fruit pulp

of *Momordica dioica* Roxb. (Cucurbitaceae). *African J. Basic and Appl. Sci.* 4(1):12-15.

102. Imaga, N.O.A. 2010. The use of phytomedicines as effective therapeutic agents in sickle cell anemia. *Sci. Res. Essays.* 5:3803-3807.

103. Jagtap, S., Satpute, R., and Mulani, R.M. 2014. Phytochemical screening, antioxidant activity and flavonoids analysis of bulb extracts of *Urginea indica* Kunth. *International Interdisciplinary Research Journal.* IV:170-186.

104. Jain, S.K. 1991. Dictionary of Indian Folk Medicine and Ethnobotany, Deep publications, New Delhi.

105. Jain, S.K. 1999. Dictionary of Ethnoveterinary Plants of India, Deep Publications, New Delhi.

106. Jamdhade, M.S., Survase, S.A., Kare, M.A. and Bhuktar, A.S. 2010. Antibacterial activity of genus *Datura* L. in Marathwada Region, Maharashtra. *Journal of Phytology.* 2(12):42-45.

107. Jamdhade, M.S., Survase, S.A., Kare, M.A. and Bhuktar, A.S. 2010. Phytochemical studies on *Datura metel* Linn. in Marathwada Region, Maharashtra. *Journal of Phytology.* 2(12):46-48.

108. Jangid, M.S. and Sharma, S.S. 2011. Poisonous plants of Modasa Taluka, District Sabarkantha (Gujarat), India. *Life Science Leaflets.* 14:462-465.

109. Jayanthi, M., Sowbala, N., Rajalakshmi, G., Kanagavalli, U. and Sivakumar, V. 2010. Study of antihyperglycemic effect of *Catharanthus roseus* in alloxan induced rats. *Int. J. Pharm Pharm Sci.* 2(Suppl.4):114-116.

110. Jehan Bakht, Azar and Mohammad Shafi. 2012. Antimicrobial activity of *Nicotiana tabacum* using different solvents extracts. *Pak. J. Bot.* 44(1):459-463.

111. Jeyaprakash, K., Ayyanar, M., Geetha, K.N. and Sekar, T. 2011. Traditional use of medicinal plants among the tribal people in Theni District (Western Ghats), Southern India. *Asian Pacific Journal of Tropical Biomedicine.* 1(supplement):520-525.

112. John De Britto, A. and Herin Sheeba Gracelin. 2011. *Datura metel* Linn. A plant with potential as antibacterial agent. *International Journal of Applied Biology and Pharmaceutical Technology.* 2(2):429-433.

113. Jummai, A.T. and Okoli, B.J. 2014. Curcin from *Jatropha curcas* seed as a potential anthelmintic. *Adv. Med. Plant Res.* 2(3):47-49.

114. Kader, J., Noor, H.M., Radzi, S.M., and Wahab, N.A.A. 2014. Antibacterial activities and phytochemical screening of the acetone extract from *Euphorbia hirta. Int. J. Med. Plants. Res.* 2(4):209-214.

115. Kalaivanan, C., Chandrasekaran, M. and Venkatesalu, V. 2014. Evaluation of antibacterial efficacy of leaves of *Cleistanthus collinus* and *Strychnos nux-vomica. International Journal of Natural Products.* 4(2):65-71.

116. Kalimuthu, K., Vijayakumar, S. and Senthilkumar, R. 2010. Antimicrobial activity of the biodiesel plant. *Jatropha curcas* L. *International Journal of Pharma and Biosciences.* 1(3):1-5.

117. Kamel, M.S., Assaf, M.H., Abe, Y., Ohtani, K., Kasai, R. and Yamasaki, K. 2001. Cardiac glycosides from *Cryptostegia grandiflora. Phytochemistry.* 58:537-542.

118. Karpreet Bhatia, Manhas, R.K., Keswal Kumar and Rani Magotra. 2014. Traditional knowledge on poisonous plants of Udhanpur district of Jammu and Kashmir, India. *Journal of Ethnopharmacology.* 152(1):207-216.

119. Karthika, S., Ravishankar, M., Mariajancyrani, J. and Chandramohan, G. 2013. Study on phytoconstituents from *Moringa oleifera* leaves. *Asian J. Plant Sci. Res.* 3(4):63-69.

120. Karuppusamy, S. 2007. Medicinal plants used by *Paliyan* tribes of Sirumalai Hills of Southern India. *Natural Product Radiance.* 6(5):436-442.

121. Katewa, S.S., Galav, P.K., Ambika Nag and Anita Jain. 2008. Poisonous plants of the Southern Aravalli hills of Rajasthan. *Indian J Traditional Knowledge* 7(2): 269-272.

122. Kawo, A.H. Mustapha, A., Abdullahi, B.A., Rogo, L.D., Gaiya, Z.A. and Kumurya, A.S. 2009. Phytochemical properties and antibacterial activities of the leaf and latex extracts of *Calotropis procera* (A.I.T.F.). *Bayero Journal of Pure and Applied Sciences.* 2(1):34-40.

123. Kiran Singh and Tafida, G.M. 2014. Antibacterial activity of *Moringa oleifera* (Lam) leaves extracts against some selected bacteria. *Int. J. Pharm Pharm Sci.* 6(9):52-54.

124. Kirtikar, K.R. and Basu, B.D. 1935. *Indian Medicinal Plants.* Vol IV. Bishen Singh, Mahendra Pal Singh, Dehradun.

125. Kirtikar, K.R. and Basu, B.D. 1999. Indian Medicinal Plants, Vol. I-IV, International Book. Distributors Book sellers and Publishers, Dehra Dun. Bishen Singh Mahendrapal Singh, New Delhi.

126. Komathi, S. and Rajalakshmi, G. 2013. Phytochemical screening and antibacterial activity of the medicinal plant – *Momordica charantia. Indian Journal of Applied Research.* 3(9):54-37.

127. Kothale, K.V., Rothe, S.P. and Pawade, P.N. 2011. Phytochemical screening of some Euphorbiaceae members. *Journal of Phytology.* 3(12):60-62.

128. Krishna, K.L., Paridhavi, M. and Patel, J.A. 2008. Review on nutritional, medicinal and pharmacological properties of *Papaya* (*Carica papaya* Linn.). *Natural Product Radiance.* 7(4):364-373.

129. Kumar Ganesan and Sharmila Banu Gani. 2013. Ethnomedical and Pharmacological potentials of *Plumbago zeylanica* L. A Review. *American Journal of Phytomedicine and Clinical Therapeutics.* 1(3):313-337.

130. Kumar, G., Karthik, L. and Bhaskara Rao, K.V. 2011. A review on pharmacological and phytochemical profile of *Calotropis gigantia* L. *Pharmacologyonline.* 1:1-8.

131. Kumar, P.S., Suresh, E., and Kalavathy, S. 2013. Review on a potential herb *Calotropis gigantia* (L.) R.Br. *Sch. Acad. J. Pharm.* 2(2):135-143.

132. Kumar, S., Pandey, S. and Pandey, A.K. 2014. *In Vitro* antibacterial, antioxidant and cytotoxic activities of *Parthenium hysterophorus* and characterization of extracts of LC-MS Analysis. *BioMed Resarch International.*

133. Kumarasamyraja, D., Jeganathan, N.S. and Manavalan, R. 2012. Pharmacological review of *Lantana camara* L. Review Article. *Int. J. Pharm. and Ind. Res.* 2(1):1-5.

134. Kumaraswamy, M., Pokharen, N., Dahal, S. and Anuradha, M. 2011. Phytochemical and antimircobial studies of leaf extract of *Euphorbia neriifolia. J. Med. Plants. Res.* 5(24):5785-5788.

135. Kushwaha, V.B. and Maurya, S. 2012. Biological utilities of *Parthenium hystroporus. J.Appl. and Nat. Sci.* 4(1):137-143.

136. Lawal, I.O., Amao, A.O. Lawal, K.O., Alamu, O.T. and Sowunmi, I.L. 2013. Phytotherapy approach for the treatement of gynaecological disorder among women in Ido local Government area of Ibadan, Oyo State, Nigeria. *J. Adv. Sci. Res.* 4(3):41-44.

137. Laximinarain Misra and Hildebert Wagener. 2007. Extraction of bioactive principles from *Mucuna pruriens* seeds. *Indian J. Biochem. Biophys.* 44:55-60.

138. Leela, C., Shashank, B. and Suresh, D. 2013. Phytochemical screening of secondary metabolites of *Euphorbia neriifolia* Linn. *Global J. Res. Med. Plants and Indigen. Med.* 2(5):292-297.

139. Leven, M., Vannen Berghe, D.A. and Mertens, F. 1979. Medicinal plants and its importance in antimicrobial activity *J. Planta Med.* 36: 311-321.

140. Loiy, E.A.H., Hasnah, M.S., Sakina, M.A.Y., Waleed, S.K. and Siddig, I.A. 2011. *In vitro* Antimicrobial activities of chloroformic, hexane and ethanolic extracts of *Citrullus lanatus* Var. citroides (Wild Melon). *J. Med. Plants Res.* 5(8): 1338-1344.

141. Mahbubur Rahman, A.H.M. and Momota Akter. 2013. Taxonomy and medicinal uses of Euphorbiaceae (Spurge) family of Rajshahi, Bangladesh. *Research in Plant Sciences.* 1(3):74-80.

142. Maheswari, J.K. (Eds). 2000. *Ethnobotany and Medicinal Plants of Indian Subcontinent.* Scientific Publisher, Jodhpur.

143. Malarkodi, E. and Manoharan, A. 2013. Antifungal activity of *Parthenium hysteroporus* L. *J. Chem. Pharm. Res.* 5(1):137-139.

144. Mandal, R. and Dhaliwal, P.K. 2007. Antifertility effect of *Melia azedarach.* Linn. (dharek) seed extract in female albino rats. *Indian J.Exp.Biol.* 45:853-860.

145. Manu Pant, Ankita Lal, Swati Rana and Anju Rani. 2012. *Plumbago zeylanica* L. : A Mini Review. *International Journal of Pharmaceutical Applications.* 3(3):399-405.

146. Maria Francis Jeffrey Bose, N., Aron, S. and Mehalingam, P. 2014. An ethnobotanical study of medicinal plants used by the Paliyars aboriginal community in Virudhunagar district, Tamilnadu, India. *Indian J.Traditional Knowledge.* 13(3):613-618.

147. Marimuthu, M., Uma Sundaram and Gurumoorthi, P. 2013. Comparative phytochemical evaluation and antibacterial activity of two different germplasm of *Mucuna. Int. J. Pharm. Pharm. Sci.* 5(2):46-51.

148. Martins, A.P., Salgueiro, L. Goncalves, M.J., Proenca Cunha, V., Vila, R., Canigueral, S., and Mazzoni, V. 2001. ESsential oil composition and antimicrobial activity of three zingiberaceae from S. Tomee principe, *J. Planta Med.* 67:580-584.

149. Matthew, K.M. 1983. The Flora of Tamilnadu Carnatic. The Rapinat Herbarium, Tiruchirapalli, Tamilandu, India.

150. McGaw, L.J. and Eloff, J.N. 2005. Screening of sixteen poisonous plants for antibacterial, anthelmintic and cytotoxic activity *In Vitra. South African J. of Bot.* 71:302-306.

151. Meera, P., Dora, P.A. and Samuet, J.K. 1999. Antibacterial effects of selected medicinal plants on the bacteria isolated from Juices. *Geobias.* 26:17-20.

152. Menghani, E., Pareek, A., Negi, R.S. and Ojha, C.K. 2011. Search for antimicrobial potentials from certain Indian medicinal plants. *Res. J. Med. Plant.* 5:295-301.

153. Mukesh Kumar, Tariq Ahmad Butt, Hussaini, S.A., Kishore Kumar, Hakimuddin Khan, Aminuddin and Samiulla, L. 2014. Ethnomedicines in the Khordha forest division of Khordha district, Odisha, India. *Int. J. Curr. Microbiol. App. Sci.* 3(1):274-280.

154. Murugalakshmi, M., Mari Selvi, J., Vallimail, M., Anitha Pushpa Rani, J. and Thangapandian, V. 2014. Preliminary phytochemical analysis and antipyretic, purgative studies of *Jatropha gossypifolia. World Journal of Pharmacy and Pharmaceutical Sciences.* 3(7):1127-1135.

155. Nampoothiri, K., Chrispal, A., Begum, A., Jasmine, S., Gopinath, K.G. and Zachariah, A. 2010. A cinical study of renal tubular dysfunction in *Cleistanthus collinus* (Oduvanthalai) Poisoning. *Clin. Toxicol.* (Phila). 48(3):193-197.

156. Naveed, M., Khan, T.A., Izhar Ali, Adil Hassan, Hamid Ali, Zaheer Ud Din, Hassan, Z., Tabassum, S., Saquib, Abdul Majid and Mujaddad Ur Rehman. 2014. *In Vitro* antibacterial activity of *Cannabis sativa* leaf extracts to some selective pathogenic bacterial strains. *Int. J. Biosci.* 4(4):65-70.

157. Nudrat, Z., Sayed and Usa Mukumdan. 2005. Medicinal and Aromatic plants of India, Part 1, In: Khan and Khanum Ukaaz Publications, Hyderabad.

158. O'Leary, S.B. 1964. Poisoning in man from eating poisonous plants. *Archives of Environmental Health.* 9:216-242.

159. Ojiako, E.N. and Okake, C.C. 2013. Determination of antioxidant of *Moringa oleifera* seed oil and its use in the production of a body cream. *Asian J. Plant Sci. Res.* 3(3): 1-4.

160. Oseni, O.A., and Akindahunsi, A.A. 2011. Some phytochemical properties and effect of fermentation on the seed of *Jatropha curcus* L. *Am. J. Food Technol.* 6:158-165.

161. Pandey, D. and Gupta, A.K. 2014. Antimicrobial activity and phytochemical analysis of *Urginea indica* from Bastar district of Chhattisgarh. *Int. J. Pharm. Sci. Rev. Res.* 26(2):273-281.

162. Pandey, N. and Barve, D. 2011. Phytochemical and pharmacological Review on *Annona squamosa* Linn. *International Journal of Pharmaceutical and Biomedical Sciences.* 2(4):1404-1412.

163. Pandikumar, P., Ayyanar, M. and Ignacimuthu, S. 2007. Medicinal plants used by *Malasar* tribes of Coimbatore district, Tamilnadu. *Indian J.Traditional Knowledge.* 6(4):579-582.

164. Parasuraman, S. and Raveendran, R. 2012. The effects of aqueous extract of *Cleistanthus collinus* (Roxb.) (Euphorbiaceae) leaves on rat blood pressure. *Pharmacognosy Research.* 4(3):178-180.

165. Parthipan, M., Aravindhan, V. and Rajendran, A. 2011. Medico - Botanical Study of Yercaud Hills in the Eastern Ghats of Tamilnadu, India. *Ancient Science of Life.* 30(4):104-109.

166. Pasayat, S.K., Sahoo, P. and Mallick, S.N. 2013. Ethno-Toxic effects of some common Angiospermic plants studied in and around Rourkela, Sundergarh, Odisha. *Life Sciences Leaflets.* 4:12-15.

167. Patil, P.J. and Ghosh, J.S. 2010. Antimicrobial activity of *Catharanthus roseus* – A Detailed Study. *Br. J. Pharm. Toxicol.* 1(1):40-44.

168. Patil, S.A. and Patil, S.B. 2011. Toxicological studies of *Momordica charantia* Linn. seed extracts in male mice. *Int. J. Morphol.* 29(4):1212-1218.

169. Poonam Agarwal. 2014. Study of some common poisonous plants in and around Fatepur, Uttar Pradesh, India. *International Journal of Pharmacy and Life Sciences.* 5(1):3223-3227.

170. Poongodi, A., Thilagavathi, S., Aravindhan, V. and Rajendran, A. 2011. Observations on some ethnomedicinal plants in Sathyamangalam forest of Erode district, Tamilnadu, India. *J.Med. Plant. Res.* 5(19): 4709-4714.

171. Prakash Ved, Somani Hema, Thomas, T.G. and Sunita, K. 2009. Mosquito larvicidal properties of latex of *Pedilanthus tithymaloids* (L.) (family : Euphorbiaceae). *J. Commun. Dis.* 41(2):129-131.

172. Prakash, M. and Sivakumar, T. 2013. A study on antibacterial activity of mangrove plant *Excoecarica agallocha. Int. J. Curr. Microbiol. App. Sci.* 2(8):260-262.

173. Prasad, H.B. 2013. Poisoning due to *Cryptostegia grandiflora* (Indian Rubbervine). *International Journal of Scientific Research.* 2(6):478-479.

174. Prasad, S.H.K.R., Swapna, N.L. and Prasad, M. 2011. Efficacy of *Euphorbia tirucalli* (L.) towards microbial activity against human pathogens. *International Journal of Pharma and Biosciences.* 2(1):B-229-N-235.

175. Prathyusha, P., Subramanian, M.S., and Sivakumar, R. 2010. Pharmacognestical studies on white and red forms of *Abrus precatorius* L. *Indian J Nat. Prod. Resour.* 1(4):476-480.

176. Priya, C.L. and Bhaskara Rao, K.N. 2011. A review on phytochemical and pharmacological profile of *Euphorbia tirucalli. Pharmacologyonline.* 2:384-390.

177. Pushpagandan, P. 1995. Ethnobiology in India: A Status Report, Government of India, New Delhi.

178. Qureshi, J.M., Bano, S., Mohammad, T. and Khan, M.A. 2001. Medicinal potential of poisonous plants of Tehsil Kahuta from district Rawalpindi, Pakistan. *Pakistan Journal of Biological Sciences.* 4:331-332.

179. Rajani Chauhan, Ruby, K.M., Aastha Shori and Jaya dwlvedi. 2012. *Plumbago zeylanica* a potent herb for various ailments : A Review. *Int. J. Pharm. Sci. Rev. Res.* 15(1):72-78.

180. Rajendran, A. and Manian, S. 2011. Herbal remedies for diabetes from the Kolli Hills, Eastern Ghats, India. *Indian J Nat. Prod. Resor.* 2:383-386.

181. Rajsakhar Saha. 2011. Pharmacognosy and Pharmacology of *Annona squamosa* – A review. *Int. J. of Pharm and Life Sci.* 2(10):1183-1189.

182. Rakhi B. Gupta., Chaudhari, P.R. and Wate, S.R. 2010. Poisonous plants in urban forest landscape of Institute Campus at Nagpur. *Ad. Plant Sci.* 23(1):293-296.

183. Ramachandra, M., Avanapu, S.R. and Shobha Rani, S. 2013. Evaluation of analgesic and anti-inflammatory activities of *Momordica charautia. Int. J. Pharm.* 3(1):176-179.

184. Ramprashed, S., Afroz, T., Mondal, B., Khan, R. and Ahmed, S. 2012. Screening of phytochemical and pharmacological activities of leaves of medicinal plant *Plumeria rubra. International Journal of Research in Pharmacy and Chemistry.* 2(4):1001-1007.

185. Rane, M.H., Sahu, N.K., Ajgoankar, S.S., Teli, N.C. and Verma, D.R. 2014. A Holistic approach on review of *Solanum virginianum* L. *Research and Review : Journal of Pharmacy and Pharmaceutical Sciences.* 3(3):1-4.

186. Rauf, A. and Muhammad, N. 2013. Phytochemical and Pharmacological evaluation of aerial parts of *Euphorbia pulcherrima* L. *Wudpecker Journal of Pharmacy and Pharmacology.* 2(2):15-20.

187. Rauf, A., Khan, A., Uddin, N. and Roohullah. 2013. Cytotoxic study of aerial parts of *Euphorbia milli* and *Euphorbia pulcherrima.*

188. Ravikumar, V.R. and Sudha, T. 2011. Phytochemical and antimicrobial studies on *Plumbago zeylanica* (L.) (Plumbaginaceae). *International Journal of Research in Pharmacy and Chemistry.* 1(2):185-188.

189. Riazullah, Iqbal Hussain and Badrullah. 2012. Phytochemical and anti-microbial activity of *Lepidium sativum* L. *J.Med. Plants Res.* 6(26): 4358-4361.

190. Rita, P. and Animesh, D.K. 2011. An updated overview on *Solanum xanthocarpum* Schrad and Wendl. *International Journal of Research in Ayurveda and Pharmacy.* 2(3):730-735.

191. Ritch -Krc, E.M., Turner, N.J. and Towers, G.H. 1996. Carrier herbal medicine and evaluation of the antimicrobial and anti-cancer activity in some frequently used remedies. *J. Ethnopharmacol.* 52:152-156.

192. Salai Senthilkumar, M.S., Vaidyanathan, D., Sivakumar, D., and Ghouse Basha, M. 2014. Diversity of ethnomedicinal plants used by Malayali tribals in Yelagiri hills of Eastern Ghats, Tamilnadu, India. *Asian J.Plant Sci. Res.* 4(1):69-80.

193. Salma, V., Rahman, M.S.M., Islam, S., Haque, N., Khatun, M., Jubair, T.A. and Paul, B.C. 2008. Mass propagation of *Rauwolfia serpentina* (L.) Benth *Pakistan Journal of Biological Sciences.* 11(9):1273-1277.

194. Salvat, A., Antonacci, L and Fortunato, R.H. 2004. Antimicrobial activity immethanoic extracts of several plant species from northern Argentina, *Phytomedicine,* 11:230-234.

195. Sandhyarani, G. and Praveen Kumar, K. 2014. Wound-healing activity of ethanolic and aqueous extracts of *Euphorbia nivulia. International Journal of Pharmacy.* 4(3):156-158.

196. Sangeetha, J. and Vijayalakshmi, K. 2011. Determination of Bioactive components of ethyl acetate fraction of *Punica granatum* rind extract. *International Journal of Pharmaceutical Sciences and Drug Research.* 3(2):116-122.

197. Sanjeeb Kalita, Gaurav Kumar, Loganathan Karthik and Kokati Venkata Bhaskara Rao. 2012. A Review on medicinal properties of *Lantana camara* Linn. *Research J. Pharm. and Tech.* 5(6):711-715.

198. Sankaranarayanan, S., Bama, P., Ramachandran, J., Kalaichelvan, P.T., Deccaraman, M., Vijayalakshmi, M., Dhamotharan, R., Dhanajeyan, B. and Sathya Bama, S. 2010. Ethnobotanical study of medicinal plants used by traditional users in Villupuram district of Tamilnadu, India. *J. Med. Plant. Res.* 4(12): 1089-1101.

199. Santos, P.R.V., Oliverira, A.C.X and Tomassini, T.C.B. 1995. Control Microbiogico de produto titoterapicos, *Rev. Farm. Bioquim,* 31:35-38.

200. Sathishkumar, D., Vamshi Sharathnath, K., Yogeswaran, P., Havani, A., Sudhakar, K., Sudha, P. and David Banji. 2010. A medicinal potency of *Momordica charantia. Internatonal Journal of Pharmaceutical Sciences Review and Research.* 1(2):95-100.

201. Sayyed, A. and Shah, M. 2014. Phytochemistry, Pharmacological and traditional uses of *Datura stramonium* L. review. *Journal of Pharmacognosy and Phytochemistry.* 2(5):123-125.

202. Scott, H.G. 1969. Poisonous plants and animals. In: food borne infections and intoxications. Edited by H.Riemann, Academic Press, New York & London, 543-564.

203. Seema Patel. 2011. Harmful and beneficial aspects of *Parthenium hysterophorus.* 3 Biotech, 1:1-9.

204. Seniya, C., Trivedia, S.S. and Verma, S.K. 2011. Antibacterial efficacy and phytochemical analysis of organic solvent extracts of *Calotropis gigantea. J. Chem. Pharm. Res.* 3(6):330-336.

205. Senthilkumar, Ganeshan, R. and Anand. 2010. Evaluation of anti-inflammatory activity of *Nerium oleander. Pharmacia.* 1(1):33-36.

206. Senthilkumar, T. and Krishnamurthy, K.V. 1993. Flora of Shevaroy Hills of Eastern Ghates. *J. Econ. Tax. Bot.* 17(3):729-748.

207. Sharma, A.K., Kharb, R. and Kaur, R. 2011. Pharmacognostical aspects of *Calotropis procera* (Ait.) R.Br. *International Journal of Pharma and Bio Sciences.* 2(3):480-488.

208. Sharma, S., Dhamija, H.K. and Parashar, B. 2012. *Jatropha curcas :* A Review. *Asian J. Res. Pharm. Sci.* 2(3):107-111.

209. Shaw, R., Siddiqui, V.A., Rajpal, Singh, V.Kr., Dey, N.R. 2009. *Cuscuta reflexa:* A double blind homoeopathic pathogenic trial. *Indian Journal of Research in Homoeopathy.* 3(3):7-13.

210. Sheeba, M., Emmanuel, S., Revathi, K. and Ignacimuthu, 2009. Wound healing activity of *Cassia occidentalis* L. in albino wistar rats. *International Journal of Integrative Biology.* 8(1):1-6.

211. Shiva Kameshwari, M.n. 2013. Chemical constituents of wild onion *Urginea indica* Kunth. Liliaceae. *Int. J. of Pharm & Life Sci.* 4(2):2414-2420.

212. Singh, B., Sharma, R.V., Vyas, G.Kr. and Sharma, P. 2011. Estimation of phytoconstituents from *Cryptostegia grandiflora* (Roxb.) R.Br. *In Vivo* and *In Vitro.* II. Antimicrobial screening. *J. Med. Plant. Res.* 5(9):1598-1605.

213. Singh, D., Jit, I. and Tyagi, S. 1999. Changing trends in acute poisoning in Chandigarh Zone : A 25 year autopsy experience from a tertiary care hospital in Northern India. *Amer. J. Forensic Med. Pathol.* 20:203-2010.

214. Singh, G.P. and Sharma, S.K. 2012. Antimicrobial evaluation of leaf extract of *Moringa oleifera* Lam. *International Research Journal of Pharmacy.* 3(4):212-215.

215. Singh, S., Singh, S., and Singh, A.P. 2013. Phytochemical investigation of different plant parts of *Calotropis gigantea. International Journal of Scientific and Research Publications.* 3(9):1-3.

216. Singh, S.K., Pandey, V.D., Singh, A. and Singh, C. 2009. Antibacterial activity of seed extracts of *Argemone mexicana* L. on some pathogenic bacterial strains. *Afr. J.Biotech.* 8(24):7077-7081.

217. Sivakumar, R. and Alagesaboopathi, C. 2007. Evaluation of anti-inflammatory properties of various forms of *Abrus precatorius L. J. Phytol. Res.* 20:207-213.

218. Sivakumar, R. and Alagesaboopathi, C. 2008. Studies on cytotoxicity and antitumor screening of red ad white forms of *Abrus precatorius L. Afr. J. Biotechnol.* 7:3984-3988

219. Sowjanya, K.M., Narendra, K., Swathi, J. and Krishna Satya, A. 2013. Phytochemical extraction and antimicrobial efficiency of crude leaf extract of medicinal plant *Cascabela thevetia. International Journal of Research in Pharmaceutical and Biomedical Sciences.* 4(2):465-470.

220. Spyker, D.A., Sauer, K., Kell, S.O. and Guerrant, R.L. 1982. A castor bean poisoning and a widely available bioassay for ricin. *Veterinary and Human Toxicology.* 24:293.

221. Sreejith, G., Jayasree, M., Latha, P.G., Suja, S.R., Shyamal, S., Shine, V.J., Anuja, G.I., Sini, S., Shikha, P., Krishnakumar, N.M., Vilash, V., Shoumya, S. and Rajasekharan, S. 2014. Hepatoprotective activity of *Oxalis corniculata* L. ethanlic extract against paracetamol induced hepatotoxicity in wistar rats and its *in vitro* antioxidant effects. *Indian J. Exp. Biol.* 52:147-152.

222. Sreejith, G., Latha, P.G., Shine, V.J., Anuja, G.I., Suja, S.R., Sini, S., Shyamal, S., Pradeep, S., Shikha, P. and Rajasekharan, S. 2010. Anti-allergic, anti-inflammatory and anti-lipidperoxidant effects of *Cassia occidentalis* Linn. *Indian J.Exp.Biol.* 48:494-498.

223. Sridhar, T.M, Josthna, P. and Naidu, C.V. 2011. Antifungal activity, phytochemical analysis of *Solanum nigrum* L. - An important antiulcer medicinal plant. *Journal of Ecobiotechnology.*3 : 11-15.

224. Srikanth, M., Swetha, T. and Veeresh, B. 2012. Phytochemistry and pharmacology of *Oxalis corniculata* Linn. A Review. *International Journal of Pharmaceutical Sciences and Research.* 3(11):4077-4085.

225. Subramanyam, D.K.S, Mooney, T., Raveendran, R. and Zachariah, B. 2003. A clinical and laboratory profile of *Cleistanthus collinus* poisoning. *J.Assoc. Physicians India.* 51:1052-1054.

226. Sudhakar, N. and Theivanai @ Vidhya, R.M. 2014. Potential medicinal properties of *Carica papaya* Linn. A mini review. *International Journal of Pharmacy and Pharmaceutical Sciences.* 6(2):1-4.

227. Suganya, R.S., Priya, K. and Sumi Roxy, B. 2012. Phytochemical screening and antibacterial activity from *Nerium oleander* and evaluate their plant mediated nanoparticle synthesis. *International Research Journal of Pharmacy.* 3(5):285-288.

228. Suman, T., and Elangomathavan, R. 2013. Bio-prospecting of *Cleistanthus collinus* and its antibacterial activity. *Asian J. Pharm. Clin. Res.* 6(Suppl. 4) 206-209.

229. Sumathi, S., Malathy, N., Dharani, B., Sivaprabha, J., Hamsa, D., Radha, P. and Padma, P.R. 2011. Antibacterial and antifungal activity of latex of *Euphorbia antiquorum*. *Afr. J. Microbiol. Res.* 5(27):4753-4756.

230. Sunil Kumar, Rashmi and Kumar, D. 2010. Evaluation of antidiabetic activity of *Euphorbia hirta* Linn. in streptozotocin induced diabetic mice. *Indian J. Nat. Prod. Reesour.* 1(2):200-203.

231. Sweta Prakash and Ashok K. Jain. 2011. Antifungal activity and preliminary phytochemical studies of leaf extract of *Solanum nigrum* Linn. *Int. J. Pharm. Pharm. Sci.* 3(Suppl. 4): 352-355.

232. Tamilselvan, N., Thirumalai, T, Shyamala, P. and David, E. 2014. A review on some poisonous plants and their medicinal values. *Journal of Acute Disease.* 85-89.

233. Thirunavukkarasu, P., Ramkumar, L. and Ramanathan, T. 2009. Anti-ulcer activity of *Excoecaria agallocha* bark on NSAID – induced Gastric ulcer in Albino rats. *Global J.Pharmacol.* 3(3):123-126.

234. Tikhomiroff, C., and Jolicoeur, M. 2002. Screening of *Catharanthus roseus* secondary metabolites by high-performance liquid chromatography. *J. Chromatogr-A.* 955:87-93.

235. Tomar, Arnit and Singh, H. 2007. Poisonous plants of Meerut district (U.P.), India. *Plant Archives.* 7(1):423-425.

236. Udayan, P.S., Satheesh George., Tushar, K.V. and Indira Balachandran. 2006. Medicinal plants used by the Malayali tribe of Servarayan Hills, Yercaud, Salem district, Tamilnadu, India. *Zoo's Print Journal* 21(4):2223-2224.

237. Ullah, R., Hussain, Z., Iqbal, Z., Hussain, J., Khan, F.U., Khan, N., Muhammed, Z., Ayaz, S., Ahad, S., Rehman, N. and Hussain, I. 2010. Traditional uses of medicinal plants in Darra Adam Khel NWFP Pakistan. *J. Med. Plants Res.* 4(17):1815-1821.

238. Umapriya, T., Rajendran, A., Aravindhan, V., Binu Thomas and Maharajan, M. 2011. Ethnobotany of Irular tribe in Palamalais Hills, Coimbatore, Tamilnadu. *Indian J Nat Prod Resour.* 2(2):250-255.

239. Uniyal, V., Bhatt, R.P., Sexena, S. and Negi, R. 2014. Phytochemical screening and anti-trichosporon activity of *Plumbago zeylanica* Linn. *Int. J. Pharm Pharm Sci.* 6(9):107-110.

240. Vaidyanathan, D., Sisubalan, N. and Ghouse Basha, M. 2014. Survey of ethnomedicinal plants and folklore studies of Malayali tribals of Vellakadai village a part of Shevaroy range in Eastern Ghats, Tamilnadu. *International Journal of REcent Scientific Research.* 5(7):1368-1380.

241. Valla Reddy, K. 2012. Acute and chronic toxicity studies of methanol extract of *Oxalis corniculata* L. in experimental animals. *Journal of Science.* 2(1):8-12.

242. Venkatanagaraju, E. and Divakar Goli. 2014. Antimicrobial activity of *Euphorbia milli* leaves extract. *Int. J.Pharm. Res. Sci.* 2(2):135-140.

243. Verma, L., Khatri, A., Kaushik, B., Patil, U.K. and Pawar, R.S. 2010. Antidiabetic activity of *Cassia occidentalis* (Linn) in normal and alloxan-induced diabetic rats. *Indian J.Pharmacol.* 42(4):224-228.

244. Vijakumar, S., Ramanathan, K. and Parimala Devi, B. 2011. *Cuscuta reflexa* Roxb. – A wonderful miracle plant in ethnomedicine. *Indian Journal of Natural Sciences.* 11(9):676-683.

245. Vijayanand, S. and Wesely, E.G. 2011. Phytochemical studies of *Melia azadirachta* and *Murraya koeingi. International Journal of Pharmaceutical Sciences and Research.* 2(5):1298-1302.

246. Viswanathan, N. and Joshi, B.S. 1983. Toxic constituent on some Indian plants. *Current Science.* 52:1-8.

247. Wakandigara, A., Nhamo, L.R.M. and Kugara, J. 2013. Chemistry of Phorbol Ester Toxicity in *Jatropha curcas* seed. A Review. *International Journal of Biochemistry Research & Review.* 3(3):146-161.

248. Waled Abdo Ahmed. 2009. Phorbol Ester as Toxic constituents of Tropical *Jatropha curcas* seed oil. *European Journal of Scientific Research.* 31(3):429-436.

249. Wannang, N.N., Ndukwe, H.C. and Nnabulfe, C. 2009. Evaluation of the analgesic properties of the *Datura metel* seeds aqueous extract. *J.Med.Plant.Res.*3(4):192-195.

250. Watt, J.M. and Breyer - Brandwijk, M.G. 1962. The medicinal and poisonous plants of Southern and Eastern Africa, Second Ed. E. and S. Livingstone, Edinburgh.

251. WHO. 2002. Traditional medicine strategy 2002-2005. WHO/EDM/TRM/2002. 1, World Health Organization, Geneva, Switzerland.

252. Yadav, J.P., Arya, V., Yadav, S., Panghal, M., Kumar, S. and Dhankhar, S. 2010. *Cassia occidentalis* L. A review on its ethnobotany, phytochemical and pharmacological profile. *Fitoterapia.* 81(4):223-230.

253. Yalla Reddy, K. 2012. Evaluation of anti-oxidants activity of whole plant of *Oxalis corniculata* L. *Inter. J. of Pharmacotherapy.* 2(1):13-17.

254. Yesmin, M.N., Uddin, S.N., Mubassara, S. and Akond, M.A. 2008. Antioxidant and antibacterial activities of *Calotropis procera* Linn. *Am-Euras. J. Agric. & Environ. Sci.* 4(5):550-553.

255. Yogesh, P., Bhat Savitha, D., Rabinarayan, A., Ashok, B.K. and Shukla, V.J. 2010. Role of shodhana on analytical parameters of *Datura innoxia* Mill and *Datura metel* Linn seeds. *International Journal of Research in Ayurveda and Pharmacy.* 1(2):249-254.

256. Yunita, F., Hanani, E. and Kristianto, J. 2012. The effect of *Carica papaya* L. leaves extract capsules on platelets count and hematocrit level in dengue fever patient. *Int. J. Med. Arom. Plants.* 2(4):573-578.

Index

B

C

D

H

I

J

K

L

M

N

O

P

Q

R

T

U

V

W

Y

Z

Made in the USA
Monee, IL
04 November 2026

67375748R00125